I0782412

1

UNDERSTANDING PROSTATE CANCER: A Comprehensive Guide to Diagnosis, Treatments and Recovery

Empowering Patients and Families Through Every Step of the Journey

By

Dr Lee W. Deleon

Dr Michael C. Owens

COPYRIGHT

All rights reserved. No part of this publication may be reproduced, distributed, or transmitted in any form or by any means, including photocopying, recording, or other electronic or mechanical methods, without the prior written permission of the publisher, except in the case of brief quotations embodied in critical reviews and certain other noncommercial uses permitted by copyright law.

<u>TABLE OF CONTENT</u>

INTRODUCTION

CHAPTER 1

Men Who Beat Prostate Cancer

CHAPTER 2

Biology of Prostate Gland

- Location, Function, Structure
- Signs and Symptoms of Prostate Problem
- Key Points on Prostate Disease
- Prostate Medical Tests

CHAPTER 3:

Causes and Risk Factors of Prostate Cancer

CHAPTER 4:

Prevention of Prostate Cancer

CHAPTER 5

Signs and Symptoms of Prostate Cancer.

FAQ (Frequently Asked Questions and Answers).

- ☐ How common is prostate cancer?
- ☐ How does prostate cancer compare with other cancers?
- ☐ Are some men more likely to be diagnosed with prostate cancer?
- ☐ How treatable is prostate cancer?
- ☐ What are the symptoms of prostate cancer? If there are no symptoms, how is prostate cancer detected?
- ☐ How is prostate cancer treated?
- ☐ What can I do to help prevent prostate cancer?
- ☐ What should you do if you or someone you love has just been diagnosed with prostate cancer

CHAPTER 7:

Categorizing Prostate Cancer.

- ☐ Staging, Grading and Grouping.

CONCLUSION

INTRODUCTION

Welcome to "Understanding Prostate Cancer: A Comprehensive Guide to Diagnosis, Treatment, and Recovery." This book is designed to be your trusted companion on the journey through prostate cancer, providing comprehensive information and guidance every step of the way. Whether you've just received a diagnosis, are exploring treatment options, or are navigating the road to recovery, this guide offers clarity, support, and empowerment.

Prostate cancer is a complex and often daunting diagnosis, but with knowledge and understanding, you can make informed decisions about your health and well-being. Written by experts in the field, this book covers everything from the basics of prostate cancer to advanced treatment options, all presented in an accessible and easy-to-understand format.

We understand that each individual's experience with prostate cancer is unique, which is why this guide emphasizes personalized care and empowerment. From understanding the different stages of prostate cancer to exploring treatment modalities tailored to your specific needs, this book equips you with the knowledge and tools to navigate your prostate cancer journey with confidence.

Whether you're a patient, caregiver, or healthcare professional, "Understanding Prostate Cancer" is here to provide the guidance and support you need to make informed decisions and achieve the best possible outcomes . Let's embark on this journey together, armed with knowledge, resilience, and hope.

CHAPTER 1

Men Who Beat Prostate Cancer

Celebrity Prostate Cancer Survivors: Stories of Hope and Resilience

In the realm of fame and fortune, even the brightest stars are not immune to the shadows cast by prostate cancer. However, amidst the daunting statistics and the uncertainty that often accompanies a diagnosis, there are tales of triumph and resilience that offer a beacon of hope to all those navigating the challenging landscape of prostate cancer.

In this chapter, we delve into the inspiring stories of famous men who have faced prostate cancer head-on and emerged victorious. From the glitz of Hollywood to the adrenaline-fueled arenas of professional sports, these celebrities have not only battled prostate cancer but have also become advocates for early detection and cutting-edge treatments.

Despite the daunting statistics, which suggest a lower survival rate once cancer spreads beyond the prostate, these stories remind us that there is reason to remain optimistic. With advancements in screening methods and innovative treatments, the outlook for men diagnosed with prostate cancer is brighter than ever before.

Join us as we explore the journeys of these celebrity survivors, whose experiences serve as a testament to the power of perseverance, the importance of early detection, and the promise of hope in the face of adversity.

The Inspiring Journey of Brian Germain: From Surgery to Success

At the age of 60, Brian Germain, a seasoned athlete with decades of martial arts experience, finally decided to schedule a long-overdue physical examination. Little did he know, this decision would uncover a life-altering diagnosis.

Having spent years training on judo and jiu-jitsu mats, Germain had neglected routine check-ups, oblivious to the importance of PSA screenings. His discovery of elevated PSA levels sent shockwaves through his world, compounded by the onset of the Covid-19 pandemic, which further delayed his medical follow-up.

After a year of waiting, Germain finally underwent radical prostatectomy in April 2021. Approaching the surgery with the same determination and discipline he brought to the mat, Germain trained rigorously, viewing his recovery as a challenge akin to preparing for a tournament. And just seven months later, against all odds, he stood victorious at the 2021 World Masters BJJ Championships in Las Vegas, clinching double gold.

But Germain's journey didn't end there. Undeterred by the challenges posed by his cancer diagnosis, he returned to the championships in 2022, once again emerging triumphant. His motto, "always ready," embodied his relentless spirit and commitment to staying prepared for any battle life threw his way.

Despite facing setbacks, including unfavorable Gleason scores and unclear margins post-surgery, Germain remains vigilant in his fight against cancer. Advocating for regular PSA screenings, he urges others not to repeat his mistake of ignoring their health until it's too late.

Now, over a year post-operation, Germain maintains a positive outlook, with his PSA levels remaining low. With the unwavering support of his wife and the serenity of their mountain retreat in North Carolina, he continues to stay in shape, embrace new challenges, and remain "always ready" for whatever life brings.

Warrior's Journey: The Resilience of Doug Maddox.

A Vietnam Veteran's Fight Against Prostate Cancer and the Power of Perseverance

Meet Doug Maddox, a true survivor whose life has been a testament to resilience and determination in the face of prostate cancer. At 76, Doug's journey is a remarkable tale of courage and strength, woven with the threads of his military service, his battles with cancer, and his unwavering optimism.

As a young man, Doug served in the U.S. Army during the Vietnam War, where he was exposed to Agent Orange, a toxic herbicide linked to prostate cancer. Despite the challenges he faced upon returning home, including raising three children as a single parent, Doug pursued various careers, traversing the country from coast to coast in pursuit of his dreams.

However, his life took an unexpected turn when he was diagnosed with prostate cancer over a decade ago. Undeterred by the daunting prospect of treatment, Doug approached his diagnosis with characteristic positivity and resilience. Despite undergoing surgery and enduring subsequent treatments, including radiation therapy and chemotherapy, Doug remained undaunted, facing each obstacle with courage and determination.

Throughout his journey, Doug has been supported by his medical team, including Dr. Ravi Parikh, who emphasizes the importance of addressing the holistic needs of cancer survivors. From managing side effects like fatigue and weight gain to maintaining bone health and mental well-being, Doug tackles each challenge head-on, armed with knowledge and determination.

Despite the ups and downs of his cancer journey, Doug remains steadfast in his outlook, embracing life with gusto and gratitude. With plans to relocate to Florida, Doug looks to the future with optimism, cherishing each moment and remaining ever grateful for the gift of life.

Doug's story serves as a beacon of hope and inspiration, reminding us all of the power of resilience, the importance of staying informed, and the value of embracing life's challenges with courage and grace.

Navigating the Path: A Stage 4 Prostate Cancer Patient's Journey

In life, there are moments that challenge us to confront our mortality, to re-evaluate our priorities, and to find strength in the face of adversity. For one man, diagnosed with stage 4 prostate cancer, these moments have become a part of his daily existence, shaping his outlook on life and his approach to living each day to the fullest.

Meet Martin Merzer, a man whose journey with cancer has been marked by resilience, introspection, and a steadfast determination to make the most out of every moment. From the initial shock of receiving his diagnosis to the ongoing battle against the disease, Martin's story is a testament to the human spirit's capacity to endure and to find hope in the midst of uncertainty. For Martin, the journey began last April when he received an email from his urologist delivering the devastating news of metastatic disease spreading throughout his body.

Despite the grim prognosis, Martin refused to let despair take hold, instead choosing to focus on raising awareness about prostate cancer and advocating for regular screenings. Throughout his treatment, Martin has been supported by his loving wife, Marion, and a network of friends and family who have rallied around him in his time of need. Together, they have navigated the ups and downs of his cancer journey, finding strength in each other and in the simple joys of everyday life.

Despite the challenges he faces, Martin remains remarkably composed and serene, embracing each day with a sense of gratitude and acceptance. While he acknowledges the uncertainties that lie ahead, he refuses to be consumed by fear or despair, choosing instead to live in the present moment and to cherish the time he has with his loved ones.As spring approaches and new life begins to bloom, Martin finds solace in the beauty of nature and the warmth of his relationships. Though the road ahead may be difficult, he is determined to face it with courage and resilience, knowing that he is surrounded by love and support every step of the way.

In the end, Martin's story is not just one of survival, but of resilience, hope, and the enduring power of the human spirit. As he continues on his journey, he serves as an inspiration to us all, reminding us to embrace each day with gratitude and to cherish the moments we have with the ones we love.

Andy Taylor's Rock and Roll Fight Against Stage 4 Prostate Cancer

Andy Taylor's Melody of Hope: A Triumph Over Stage 4 Prostate Cancer

In 2018, Andy Taylor, the iconic guitarist of Duran Duran, confronted a formidable adversary: stage 4 prostate cancer. At 62, the diagnosis shook him to the core, but Taylor resolved to confront the challenge head-on with unwavering determination.

Stage 4 prostate cancer presented a formidable foe, with cancer cells spreading beyond the prostate to other parts of Taylor's body. Despite the daunting prognosis, Taylor refused to surrender to despair. He embarked on a quest to explore treatments that could combat the cancer's advance and offer him a fighting chance at survival.

Facing the gravity of his condition, Taylor maintained his resilience, though the severity of his illness became evident as reports hinted at him receiving end-of-life care. The aggressive nature of higher-grade cancers underscored the urgency of his battle against the disease.

Amidst the darkness, a ray of hope emerged when Taylor discovered lutetium-

177, a revolutionary radiation therapy. This groundbreaking treatment sparked a remarkable transformation, breathing new life into Taylor's once-diminished spirit. After just two rounds of lutetium-177, he experienced a miraculous improvement in his health.

Taylor's journey from feeling like the "walking dead" to embracing life once more captivated audiences worldwide. His appearance on "Lorraine" in September 2023 served as a testament to his resilience and determination in overcoming adversity.

Lutetium-177, hailed as a game-changer in the fight against advanced prostate cancer, offered Taylor and countless others a glimmer of hope amid their darkest days. While it wasn't a cure, this innovative therapy symbolized a beacon of possibility for cancer patients everywhere, reminding them that hope and resilience can prevail even in the face of the most daunting challenges.

Sheffler Strong: Triumph Over Prostate Cancer

In March 2021, Pat Sheffler's life took an unexpected turn when a routine physical revealed concerning news – his PSA levels were alarmingly high. At age 53, Pat, a vibrant multi-sport athlete, was diagnosed with Stage 3 prostate cancer, sending shockwaves through his world. However, Pat's unwavering determination and the unwavering support of his family propelled him on a journey of resilience and hope.

Faced with a daunting diagnosis, Pat embarked on a relentless quest for the best treatment options. Through extensive research and consultation with medical experts, he found himself at the forefront of a groundbreaking clinical trial at UCSD, led by PCF-researcher Dr. Rana McKay. The trial offered a glimmer of hope, aiming to test the efficacy of potent hormonal therapies in combating advanced prostate cancer.

Pat's journey was not just one of medical treatment; it was a testament to the power of positivity and unwavering support. Surrounded by a loving family and a community rallying behind him, Pat faced each challenge with an indomitable spirit. His son, Brandon, adorned in a shirt emblazoned with "Positive Vibes" and "Sheffler Strong," epitomized the unwavering support that buoyed Pat through his darkest days.

As Pat underwent surgery and grueling treatments, his resilience never wavered. Despite the physical toll, he continued to embrace life with unwavering optimism and determination. His commitment to staying active, both physically and mentally, became a beacon of inspiration for all those around him.

Months passed, and Pat's perseverance paid off. A year after surgery, he received the long-awaited news – his PSA levels were undetectable, and his testosterone was rising back to normal. It was a triumph not only for Pat but for the countless individuals rooting for his success.

For Pat Sheffler, his journey through prostate cancer was more than a battle against a disease; it was a testament to the power of positivity, resilience, and unwavering support. As he continues to embrace life with open arms, Pat's story serves as a beacon of hope for all those facing their own medical challenges. With determination and a positive mindset, anything is possible – even triumphing over adversity and emerging stronger on the other side.

Love Story of Milton and Shawni Wilborn

In a heart-wrenching yet inspiring tale of love and perseverance, the story of Milton and Shawni Wilborn unfolds, entwined with the challenges of prostate cancer. Their journey began over three decades ago in the corridors of high school, where their paths crossed but destiny had other plans. Despite their mutual desire, circumstances kept them apart until the digital age reunited them through Facebook, reigniting a flame that had never truly died.

Their love story took a tumultuous turn when they embarked on a new life together in Virginia. Milton, a dedicated father of two, had just celebrated his 45th birthday when prostate issues surfaced unexpectedly. Despite his commitment to fitness, subtle signs hinted at an underlying health concern. With unwavering support, Shawni stood by his side as they navigated the complexities of diagnosis and treatment.

Their journey became a testament to the importance of awareness and proactive health management. Milton's age at diagnosis, 45, underscored the significance of early detection in combating prostate cancer. As the couple grappled with the physical and emotional toll of chemotherapy, they found solace in their shared faith and commitment to each other.

Despite the challenges, their love endured, and they exchanged vows in 2017, with Shawni serving as Milton's unwavering pillar of strength and support. Their bond deepened as they confronted each obstacle together, drawing strength from their love and the resilience of their shared journey.

Through their experiences, Milton and Shawni emerged as advocates for education and empowerment, sharing their story to raise awareness about prostate cancer. Milton's years of survival after treatment, a testament to his courage and determination, offered hope to others facing similar battles.

As Milton's journey continued, marked by milestones and setbacks alike, Shawni remained by his side, their love shining brightly through the darkest of times. Despite the challenges, they cherished each moment together, finding joy in the simple pleasures of life and the enduring bond they shared.

Milton's legacy lives on, a testament to the transformative power of love and resilience in the face of adversity. His years of survival after treatment stand as a beacon of hope, inspiring others to prioritize their health and cherish the precious moments they have with their loved ones. Through their story, Milton and Shawni remind us all of the profound impact of love and the strength it provides in our greatest trials.

CHAPTER 2.
BIOLOGY OF PROSTATE GLAND

The prostate, often confused with "prostrate," is a small, resilient gland roughly the size of a ping-pong ball. Positioned deep within the groin, nestled between the base of the penis and the rectum, it plays a crucial role in reproduction. This gland contributes a portion of seminal fluid, which combines with sperm from the testes to facilitate their movement and survival.

Understanding the prostate's anatomy, including its normal development and function, its precise location, and its adjacent structures, is vital for comprehending the onset and progression of prostate cancer. Whether through the growth of cancer cells or the side effects of treatments, prostate cancer profoundly impacts a man's quality of life over time.

Location of the Prostate

The prostate sits deep inside the groin. The seminal vesicles are rabbit-eared structures that sit on top of the prostate and store and secrete a large portion of the ejaculate.

The neurovascular bundle is a collection of nerves and blood vessels that run along each side of the prostate, and helps to control erectile function. In some men, these nerves run a short distance away from the prostate, but in others, they attach to the prostate itself. Their precise location doesn't impact prostate function or contribute to prostate cancer when it occurs.

The bladder is like a balloon that gets larger as it fills with urine. The urethra, a narrow tube that connects to the bladder, runs through the middle of the prostate and along the length of the penis, carrying both urine and semen out of the body. It is the hose that drains the bladder.

The rectum, which sits right behind the prostate, is the lower end of the intestines and connects to the anus.

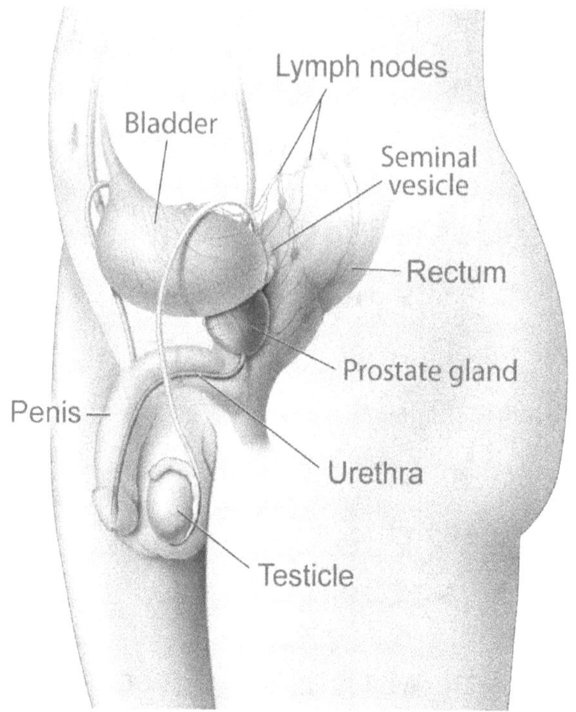

The Functions of Prostate Gland

The role of the prostate gland in human physiology is primarily linked to fertility, although it is not essential for survival. Below are the key functions associated with the prostate:

1. Semen Production:

- The prostate gland plays a crucial role in producing prostatic fluid, which contributes to semen.

- Approximately 20–30% of the total semen volume is derived from the prostate, with the seminal vesicles (50–65%) and testicles (5%) also contributing.

- Prostatic fluid contains various components essential for creating an optimal environment for sperm cells, such as enzymes, zinc, and citric acid.

- Notably, the enzyme prostate-specific antigen (PSA) aids in thinning and liquefying semen, facilitating sperm movement.

- The fluid component of semen assists sperm in traversing the urethra and surviving the journey towards fertilization, thereby supporting reproduction.

2. pH Regulation:

- ☐ Prostatic fluid maintains a slightly acidic pH, which is essential for sperm function.
- ☐ However, semen as a whole tends to be alkaline due to contributions from other components, counteracting the natural acidity of the vagina and safeguarding sperm from potential damage.

3 Ejaculation Regulation:

- ☐ During ejaculation, the prostate undergoes contractions, releasing prostatic fluid into the urethra.

- This fluid combines with sperm cells and seminal vesicle fluid to form semen, which is subsequently expelled from the body.

- Contraction of the prostate during ejaculation also serves to close off the passage between the bladder and urethra, facilitating the rapid expulsion of semen.

- As a result, simultaneous urination and ejaculation are typically not possible under normal anatomical conditions.

4. Hormone Metabolism:

- The proper functioning of the prostate relies on male sex hormones, known as androgens, particularly testosterone.

- Within the prostate gland, an enzyme called 5-alpha reductase plays a crucial role in converting testosterone into dihydrotestosterone (DHT), a biologically active form of the hormone.

☐ DHT is essential for normal prostate development and function, particularly during the male developmental stages, where it contributes to the emergence of secondary sexual characteristics like facial hair growth.

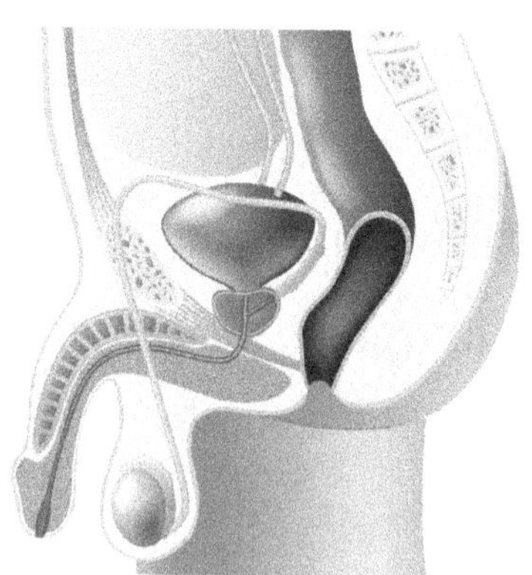

Structure Of Prostate Gland

The prostate gland's structure consists of several layers enclosed within a capsule of connective tissue, imparting a resilient texture to the gland. Medical experts typically divide the prostate into four distinct zones, analogous to the layers of an onion, arranged from the outermost to the innermost regions:

1. Anterior Fibromuscular Zone (AFZ): Comprising muscle and fibrous tissues, this zone is known as the anterior fibromuscular zone in medical terminology.

2. Peripheral Zone: (PZ) Predominantly located at the rear of the gland, this area houses the majority of the glandular tissue.

3. Central Zone (CZ): Encompassing the ejaculatory ducts, this zone constitutes approximately 25% of the prostate's overall mass.

4. Transition Zone (TZ): Surrounding the urethra, this segment of the prostate is the only part that undergoes continuous growth throughout an individual's life.

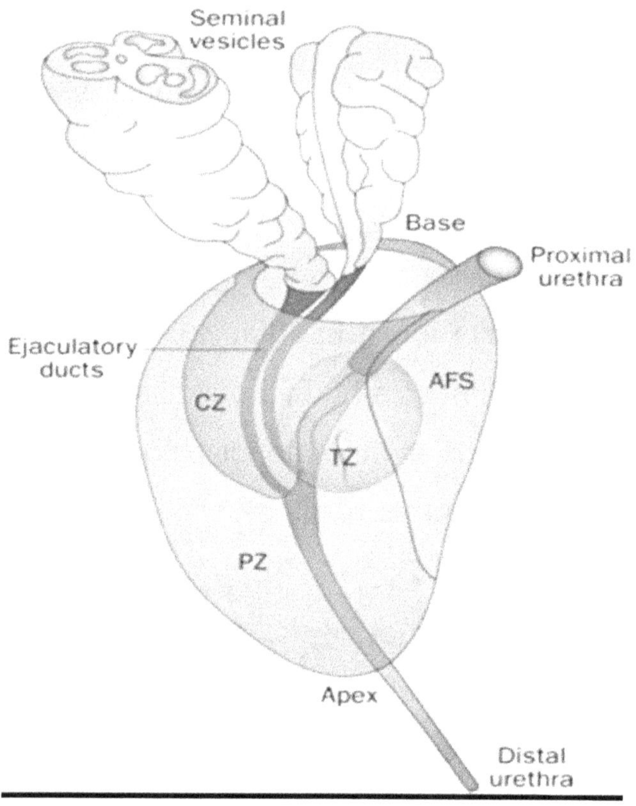

Anterior Fibromuscular Zone (AFZ):

Peripheral Zone: (PZ)

Central Zone (CZ):

Transition Zone (TZ):

Signs and Symptoms of Prostate Problems

Conditions related to the prostate often manifest in urinary or bladder difficulties. **These symptoms may encompass:**

- Challenges with bladder control, leading to frequent visits to the bathroom.
- Urgent or sudden urges to urinate, sometimes resulting in the release of only a small amount of urine.
- Struggles initiating the urine stream, or interruptions and restarts during urination.
- A feeble or narrow urine flow.

Prostate problems can also trigger issues with sexual function, urinary infections, bladder stones, or in severe instances, kidney malfunction. If an individual experiences complete inability to urinate, seeking immediate medical attention is imperative.

It's advisable to consult a healthcare professional if any of the subsequent symptoms are observed:

- ☐ Pain during urination or post-ejaculation.
- ☐ Discomfort in the penis, scrotum, or perineal area.
- ☐ Presence of blood in the urine.
- ☐ Severe abdominal pain.
- ☐ Weak urine stream or dribbling following urination.
- ☐ Onset of fever, chills, or generalized body aches.
- ☐ Difficulties managing bladder function, such as delays in urination or incomplete bladder emptying.
- ☐ Detection of abnormal odor or color in the urine.

Key Points On Prostate Conditions

1. Prostate Cancer:

- Most common cancer in males after skin cancer, affecting 1 in 8 males during their lifetime.
- Typically diagnosed around age 66.
- Screening is optional and should be based on age and risk factors, considering potential risks.

2. Prostatitis:

- Common inflammation of the prostate, most prevalent in males under 50.
- Around 10-15% of males in the U.S. will experience prostatitis.
- Acute prostatitis is sudden and bacterial, while chronic prostatitis lasts over 3 months.

3. **Enlarged Prostate (BPH**):

- ☐ Common in males over 50.
- ☐ Enlargement can lead to urethral constriction, causing urinary difficulties.
- ☐ Symptoms include difficulty urinating and potential urinary retention, necessitating urgent medical attention.

Prostate Medical Tests

Medical professionals can diagnose problems with the prostate using various types of prostate exams.

Common prostate exams include:

- **Prostate-specific antigen (PSA):** Blood tests can assess the levels of this PSA. High levels indicate an increased risk of prostate cancer.

- **Digital rectal examination**: During this exam, the doctor inserts a finger into the rectum and feels the prostate to detect lumps, nodules, and signs of cancer
- **Prostate biopsy:** If a doctor suspects cancer, they can take a small sample of prostate tissue for testing. To do this, they insert a needle into the prostate via the rectum.
- **Prostate ultrasound:** Doctors may refer to this as a transrectal ultrasound. During the procedure, the medical professional inserts a probe into the rectum, positioning it close to the prostate. Doctors usually carry out biopsies with guidance from an ultrasound.
- **Prostate MRI:** This can show prostate anatomy in great detail,

including identifying areas suspicious for cancer. New technology allows targeting of these areas through an MRI-ultrasound fusion biopsy.

CHAPTER 3
CAUSES AND RISK FACTORS OF PROSTATE CANCER.

If you or someone close to you has received a prostate cancer diagnosis, you might be searching for answers, wondering about the cause. What led to this situation? Could anything have been done differently to prevent it? The explanation is straightforward, though not entirely satisfying: medical experts and researchers currently lack precise knowledge of the exact causes.

However, four primary risk factors have been identified: racial background, family history, age and lifestyle.

Lifestyle, such as: smoking, obesity, and potentially excessive calcium intake, appear to contribute to more aggressive forms of prostate cancer. However, these factors are also associated with various other health issues. Individuals with underlying health conditions may experience worse outcomes when dealing with any illness.

One of the primary underlying factors, which we have limited influence over, is our genetic makeup. At conception, genetic material from both parents combines to form a unique genetic profile containing all the necessary information for the development of an individual. However, sometimes this genetic code contains variations that are associated with certain illnesses later in life.

Specifically, mutations in genes like BRCA1 and BRCA2 are known to be linked to certain familial cancers. Families with a history of these cancers can undergo genetic screening. However, inherited genetic mutations are estimated to contribute to only 5% to 10% of prostate cancer cases.

Acquired mutations are another type of genetic alterations that occur after your conception. These changes happen as your cells continually regenerate, with each cell division presenting a possibility for genetic errors during the copying process. While the precise factors influencing this process are not fully understood, various elements such as body chemistry, hormone levels, exposure to toxins, dietary habits, physical activity, and radiation exposure (e.g., from the sun) are implicated in the occurrence of acquired gene mutations.

In essence, the answer is both straightforward and complex, echoing the advice often provided by healthcare professionals for maintaining overall health: prioritize a balanced diet, regular exercise, and sufficient rest to reduce the risk of prostate cancer. Additionally, it's essential to adhere to a proactive screening schedule for prostate cancer as you age.

Prostate Cancer Risk Factors

Three primary risk factors are widely recognized for prostate cancer:

1. Advancing age
2. Family history, including genetic predisposition
3. African American ethnicity

As men grow older, their susceptibility to prostate cancer notably escalates, with approximately 60% of diagnoses occurring in those aged over 65. Consequently, initiating discussions with a healthcare provider regarding prostate-specific antigen (PSA) screening upon reaching middle age holds significant importance.

Genetic inheritance plays a substantial role in prostate cancer, with genetics accounting for 58% of its incidence.

Individuals with a close family member diagnosed with prostate cancer may face double the risk, while those with two or more affected relatives may have nearly quadruple the risk, particularly if the relatives were diagnosed before age 60. Additionally, a heightened risk of prostate cancer may exist in individuals with a family history of other cancers like breast, ovarian, colon, or pancreatic cancer.

Unraveling the genetic complexities of cancer has revealed specific genes, such as BRCA2, that can elevate prostate cancer risk when certain mutations are present. Consequently, individuals harboring these genetic alterations may require tailored screening protocols.

Prostate cancer affects Black men disproportionately, with one in six facing a diagnosis in their lifetime, compared to one in eight white men. Moreover, Black men are more than twice as likely to succumb to the disease. They tend to receive diagnoses at younger ages and with more aggressive forms of the illness.

The higher mortality rate among Black men with prostate cancer is attributed, in part, to disparities in healthcare access, insurance coverage, PSA screening availability, suitable treatment options, and follow-up care, along with various socioeconomic factors.

Ongoing research endeavors aim to ascertain potential biological disparities in prostate cancer among Black men, with the goal of enhancing treatment outcomes. However, it's vital to recognize that not all Black men will develop prostate cancer, and early detection significantly improves the likelihood of effective management and cure.

Additional factors contributing to the risk of prostate cancer diagnosis and poorer prognosis include social and environmental influences, notably dietary habits characterized by low vegetable intake and high consumption of processed meats and saturated fats, along with lifestyle choices. Overweight or obese men face an increased likelihood of developing aggressive prostate cancer forms. Studies indicate that obese individuals tend to experience prolonged and more challenging post-surgery recovery, coupled with a heightened risk of prostate cancer mortality.

Research in the past few years has shown that dietary factors might decrease the chances of developing prostate cancer, reduce the likelihood of having a prostate cancer recurrence, or help slow the progression of the disease.

Risk and Other Prostate Conditions

Distinguishing between aggressive and slow-growing prostate cancers has revealed various risk factors unique to each subtype. For instance, while smoking doesn't seem to contribute to low-risk prostate cancer, it may heighten the risk of aggressive forms.

Similarly, inadequate consumption of vegetables, particularly those from the broccoli family, correlates with an increased risk of aggressive prostate cancer but not with low-risk cases. Although body mass index (BMI) isn't associated with an overall prostate cancer diagnosis, obese individuals are more prone to aggressive disease, likely due to factors such as dilution of PSA in a larger blood volume.

Additionally, factors like tall height, sedentary lifestyle, high calcium intake, Black race, family history, and exposure to Agent Orange have been linked to aggressive prostate cancer.

There's a common misconception regarding the relationship between non-cancerous prostate conditions and the risk of prostate cancer. While these conditions may manifest symptoms similar to those of prostate cancer and warrant evaluation by a physician, there's no evidence to suggest that having either of the following conditions increases a man's risk of developing prostate cancer.

One such condition is Benign Prostatic Hyperplasia (BPH), characterized by a non-cancerous enlargement of the prostate. This enlargement can lead to the compression of the urethra, causing difficulty and often pain during urination.

Prostatitis, an infection in the prostate, is the most common cause of urinary tract infections in men. Most treatment strategies are designed to relieve the symptoms of prostatitis, which include fever, chills, burning during urination, or difficulty urinating.

There have been links between inflammation of the prostate and prostate cancer in several studies. This may be a result of being screened for cancer just by having prostate-related symptoms, and currently, this is an area of controversy.

More Myths and Non-Risks

Sexual Activity: Contrary to rumors, high levels of sexual activity or frequent ejaculation do not increase prostate cancer risk. In fact, studies indicate that men reporting more frequent ejaculations may have a reduced risk of developing prostate cancer.

Vasectomy: Previous beliefs linking vasectomy to an increased risk of prostate cancer have been debunked.

Medications (aspirin, statins): Recent research suggests that aspirin intake may reduce the risk of prostate cancer by 10-15%. This reduction could be attributed to various factors such as different screening practices, inflammation reduction, or other unknown factors. Similarly, statins, typically used to lower cholesterol, have been associated with a reduced risk of aggressive prostate cancer in some studies. However, it's important to note that neither aspirin nor statins are recommended solely for the prevention or treatment of prostate cancer.

Alcohol: There is no established direct correlation between alcohol consumption and prostate cancer risk.

Supplements (Vitamin E, selenium): Recent studies have not demonstrated any beneficial effect of vitamin E or selenium (in the studied formulations) in preventing prostate cancer.

CHAPTER 4
PREVENTION OF
PROSTATE CANCER

The primary aim is to prevent the onset of prostate cancer altogether. While significant strides have been made and both genetic and environmental risk factors for prostate cancer have been identified, conclusive recommendations on overall prostate cancer prevention are lacking due to insufficient evidence.

Nevertheless, there are several measures men can adopt to potentially lower their risk. **Dietary adjustments and lifestyle** modifications have demonstrated efficacy in reducing the risk of developing aggressive or fatal prostate cancer, as well as in slowing down prostate cancer progression post-diagnosis. These lifestyle changes can also contribute to improved longevity and quality of life for men living with prostate cancer.

Understanding the causative factors of prostate cancer is pivotal in prevention strategies. Three major factors influence the risk of developing prostate cancer:

1. <u>Age</u> Prostate cancer diagnosis typically occurs around the age of 66 in the U.S. While rare in men under 50, the risk increases with age. For instance, the probability stands at 1 in 457 for men under 50, 1 in 55 for those aged 50-59, 1 in 19 for ages 60-69, and 1 in 11 for ages 70 and older.

2. **Race**: In the U.S., Black men face a significantly higher likelihood of developing prostate cancer, with about a 70% chance, and are more than twice as likely to succumb to it.

3. Family History: Men with a family history of prostate cancer, especially if a close relative like a father or brother has been affected, may have double the risk compared to those without such a history. The risk escalates further if the cancer was diagnosed at an earlier age or multiple family members are affected.

It's crucial to discuss any family history of not only prostate cancer but also other cancers like breast, ovarian, colon, pancreatic, endometrial, or multiple other cancers with a healthcare provider.

While some risk factors are beyond modification, there are numerous proactive steps men can take to potentially lower their risk of developing aggressive prostate cancer or experiencing a recurrence.

10 Tips for Prostate Cancer Prevention

1. Adopt an "anti-inflammatory diet," low in red meat, sugar, processed foods, and dairy products, and high in foods that fight inflammation, such as brightly-colored vegetables.

2. Eat fewer calories and exercise more so that you maintain a healthy weight. Vigorous exercise, within the bounds of safety for your personal physical fitness level, has been

shown to reduce a man's chance of developing lethal forms of prostate cancer. Obesity is linked to increased risk of fatal prostate cancer and of prostate cancer recurrence.

3. Watch your calcium intake. Very high amounts of calcium may increase risk of aggressive prostate cancer. Try to get most of your calcium from plant-based food sources (e.g., almonds, tofu, leafy greens) rather than supplements, unless your doctor has advised otherwise.

4. Swap red meat for plant-based protein and fish. Saturated fat in red meat is a cause of inflammation, which is associated with cancer and other chronic diseases. Avoid trans

fatty acids (e.g., margarine, packaged baked goods).

5. Incorporate cooked tomatoes (prepared with olive oil), which may be beneficial, and cruciferous vegetables (like broccoli and cauliflower) into many of your weekly meals.

6. Avoid smoking for many reasons. Drink alcohol in moderation, if at all.

7. Seek medical treatment for stress, high blood pressure, diabetes, high cholesterol, and depression. Treating these conditions may save your life and will improve your survivorship with prostate cancer.

8. Avoid over-supplementation with megavitamins. While a multivitamin is not likely to be harmful, you probably don't need it if you follow a healthy diet with lots of fruits, vegetables, whole grains, fish, and healthy oils. Ask your doctor about herbal supplements, as some may harm you or interfere with treatment.

9. Relax and enjoy life. Studies have shown that the stress hormone cortisol can interfere with cancer cell death. Reducing stress in the workplace and home will improve your survivorship and lead to a longer, happier life.

10. For men age 45 or older (40 or older for Black men or those with a family history of prostate cancer),

discuss the risks and benefits of screening with a PSA test and, if indicated, a rectal examination, with your doctor.

CHAPTER 5

SIGNS AND SYMPTOMS OF PROSTATE CANCER.

After receiving a recent diagnosis of prostate cancer, you might be wondering whether there were any indications or symptoms you overlooked earlier. So, what are the indicators of prostate cancer? Regrettably, there are typically no early signs for prostate cancer. The developing tumor doesn't exert pressure on surrounding areas to provoke pain, resulting in many years of silent progression of the disease. This underscores the significance of prostate cancer screening for all men and their loved ones.

Should I Undergo Screening?

You may have encountered conflicting viewpoints regarding prostate cancer screening. What exactly does the test entail? Is it truly necessary? Surprisingly, there's ongoing debate regarding the suitability of routine annual prostate cancer screening, primarily because prostate cancer often progresses slowly. In fact, it's feasible to lead a healthy life while having prostate cancer that is being closely monitored without active treatment, a practice known as Active Surveillance. However, certain cases of prostate cancer pose an immediate threat and necessitate treatment.

The majority of prostate cancers are detected early through screening.

Early-stage prostate cancer typically does not present symptoms. However, in some cases, symptoms may include:

Difficulty urinating, such as a slow or weak urinary stream, frequent urination (especially at night), or the presence of blood in the urine or semen.

In addition to the above symptoms, advanced prostate cancer may lead to other manifestations, including:

- Erectile dysfunction (ED)
- Pain in various areas like the hips, back (spine), or chest (ribs), indicating cancer spread to the bones.
- Weakness, numbness in the legs or feet, or loss of bladder or bowel

control due to spinal cord compression by cancer.

☐ Weight loss and extreme fatigue.

While these symptoms can be associated with prostate cancer, they are often caused by other conditions. For instance, benign prostatic hyperplasia (BPH), a non-cancerous prostate enlargement, commonly leads to difficulties in urination.

Nevertheless, it's crucial to inform your healthcare provider if you experience any of these symptoms to undergo appropriate evaluation and potential treatment. Some individuals may require further testing to assess for prostate cancer.

When to Get Checked for Prostate Cancer

Take initiative as you reach middle age (between 40 to 50 years), take proactive steps by consulting your doctor regarding establishing a suitable schedule for prostate cancer screenings tailored to your individual risk factors and family medical history.

The timing of initiating screenings is contingent upon specific risk factors, which vary among different demographic groups. These are considerations to take into account when devising a proactive plan for prostate cancer screenings that suits your needs.

Ask yourself:

- [ ] What is your age?
- [ ] Is there a family history of prostate, ovarian, breast, colon, or pancreatic cancers among your relatives, both male and female?
- [ ] Do you have African ancestry?

Be vigilant for warning signs. Unfortunately, prostate cancer often does not present early warning signs. Since a growing prostate tumor typically does not exert pressure to cause pain, the disease may remain asymptomatic for many years. However, there are specific signs and symptoms that warrant discussion with your doctor.

In certain instances, particularly in advanced stages, prostate cancer can manifest symptoms such as:

- A need to urinate frequently, especially at night, sometimes urgently
- Difficulty starting or holding back urination
- Weak, dribbling, or interrupted flow of urine
- Painful or burning urination
- Difficulty in having an erection
- A decrease in the amount of fluid ejaculated
- Painful ejaculation
- Blood in the urine or semen
- Pressure or pain in the rectum
- Pain or stiffness in the lower back, hips, pelvis, or thighs

Many types of cancer are much more prevalent in people with certain genetic mutations, so if you learn that a blood relative is experiencing one of these cancers—even if they are the first or only relative diagnosed—you should start a conversation with your doctor about ramping up your own screening regimen or considering genetic testing.

Watch for breast, ovarian, prostate, pancreatic, and colorectal cancers in particular, as these are known to arise in families sharing certain genetic mutations.

Genetic tests are fairly new, but they represent an opportunity to get ahead of cancer.

If your family has traditionally kept quiet about health issues, you now have an opportunity to change that pattern and enhance the well-being of your entire family. Detecting prostate cancer early increases the likelihood of successful treatment, and some low-risk cancers may not require immediate intervention.

However, early signs and symptoms are often absent, leaving many men unaware of any potential problems until they undergo routine screening and receive a cancer diagnosis. Consult with your doctor to develop a personalized screening strategy that suits your needs.

Prostate Cancer FAQ (Frequently Asked Questions)

How common is prostate cancer?

- ☐ Prostate cancer ranks as the most prevalent non-skin cancer among men in the United States and stands as the fourth most common tumor diagnosed globally.
- ☐ In the U.S., statistics indicate that 1 in 8 men will receive a prostate cancer diagnosis within his lifetime.
- ☐ Among Black men, the likelihood increases to 1 in 6, with a stark reality of being over twice as likely to succumb to the disease.

☐ By the year 2024, projections suggest that over 299,000 men in the U.S. will confront a diagnosis of prostate cancer, with more than 35,000 succumbing to the illness. This translates to a new case diagnosed every two minutes and a prostate cancer-related death every 15 minutes.

☐ Remarkably, the probability of a man developing prostate cancer surpasses the combined likelihood of developing colon, kidney, melanoma, and stomach cancers.

How does prostate cancer compare with other cancers?

- ☐ Prostate cancer holds the distinction of being the most prevalent non-skin cancer among men in the U.S., and globally, it ranks fourth in terms of diagnosis frequency.

- ☐ The probability of a man developing prostate cancer outweighs the collective likelihood of developing colon, kidney, melanoma, and stomach cancers combined.

Are some men more likely to be diagnosed with prostate cancer?

- The risk of prostate cancer diagnosis escalates notably after reaching the age of 50, with approximately 6 out of 10 cases diagnosed in men aged 65 and above.

- Black men face a heightened risk, with 1 in 6 expected to receive a prostate cancer diagnosis and facing more than double the mortality rate compared to other demographic groups. Further insights into prostate cancer among Black men can be found here.

- Notably, prostate cancer ranks among the most heritable of major human cancers, with genetic factors contributing to an estimated 57% of the risk associated with the disease.

How Treatable Is Prostate Cancer?

More than 80% of all prostate cancers are detected when the cancer is in the prostate or the region around it, so treatment success rates are high compared to most other types of cancer in the body. The 5-year overall survival rates in the United States for men diagnosed with local or regional prostate cancer exceed 99%. In other words, the chances of men dying from their prostate cancer is generally low. However, prostate cancer comes in many forms, and some prostate cancers can be aggressive even when they first appear to be confined to the prostate.

What are the symptoms of prostate cancer? If there are no symptoms, how is prostate cancer detected?

What are the symptoms of prostate cancer?

If the cancer is caught at its earliest stages, most men will not experience any symptoms. Some men, however, will experience symptoms such as frequent, hesitant, or burning urination, difficulty in having an erection, or pain or stiffness in the lower back, hips or upper thighs.

Because these symptoms can also indicate the presence of other diseases or disorders, men who experience any of these symptoms will undergo a thorough work-up to determine the underlying cause of the symptoms.

If there are no symptoms, how is prostate cancer detected?

Screening for prostate cancer can be performed in a physician's office. Prostate specific antigen (PSA) testing is the current test of choice for prostate cancer screening. During a PSA test, a small amount of blood is drawn from the arm, and the level of PSA is measured. When there's a problem with the prostate—such as the development and growth of prostate cancer—more PSA is released. This can be the first indicator of prostate cancer. More testing, such as digital rectal exam (DRE), imaging, and, ultimately, a biopsy, is required to confirm a diagnosis.

How is prostate cancer treated?

There are a wide variety of treatment options available for men with prostate cancer, including surgery, radiation therapy, hormone therapy and chemotherapy, any or all of which might be used at different times depending on the stage of disease and the need for treatment.

Consultation with all three types of prostate cancer specialists—a urologist, a radiation oncologist and a medical oncologist—will offer the most comprehensive assessment of the available treatments and expected outcomes. For men with advanced disease or an increased risk due to family history or lifestyle, precision treatments based on genetic screening may be recommended.

How Can I Lower My Risk of Prostate Cancer?

1. Maintain a healthy weight by reducing calorie intake and increasing physical activity.
2. Limit consumption of fat derived from red meat and dairy products.
3. Monitor calcium intake, avoiding excessive supplementation beyond the recommended daily allowance of 1,200 mg.

4. Incorporate fish into your diet for its omega-3 fatty acids, while avoiding trans fatty acids found in products like margarine.

5. Include cooked tomatoes with olive oil, cruciferous vegetables like broccoli and cauliflower, soy-based foods, and green tea in your meals.

6. Quit smoking and drink alcohol in moderation, if at all.

7. Address medical conditions such as stress, high blood pressure, diabetes, high cholesterol, and depression to enhance overall health and survivorship.

8. Use caution with megavitamin supplementation, opting for a balanced diet rich in fruits, vegetables, whole grains, fish, and healthy oils. Consult

your doctor regarding herbal supplements.

9. Prioritize relaxation and enjoyment to reduce stress levels, fostering a longer and happier life.

10. Men aged 45 and older (or 40 and older for Black men or those with a family history of prostate cancer) should discuss the benefits and risks of prostate cancer screening, including PSA tests and rectal examinations, with their healthcare provider.

What should you do if you or someone you love has just been diagnosed with prostate cancer?

There are many options for treatment at all stages of prostate cancer. If you are diagnosed with prostate cancer, make sure to get on the "right track": that is, the right team, the right tests, and the right treatments, right from the start.

CHAPTER 6
Screening, Diagnosis and Treatment Of Prostate Cancer

Cancer can be a scary thought, but modern medical advancements offer powerful tools for screening, and one thing we know for sure: catching cancer early can save lives. Typically, prostate cancer screening commences with a prostate-specific antigen (PSA) test, involving the extraction of a small blood sample from the arm to measure the level of PSA, a protein produced by the prostate. Controversy surrounds the risks and benefits of prostate cancer screening, leading to evolving recommendations over time.

Detecting cancer in its early stages greatly increases the chances of successful treatment, if treatment is warranted. For prostate cancer, the survival rate is promising, with 99% of men diagnosed at an early stage living five years or longer after diagnosis. Early detection also grants individuals the option to monitor slow-growing cancer rather than opting for immediate treatment. While there are no inherent risks associated with screening, timing is a critical factor to consider. So, when should you start screening for prostate cancer? Most experts advise discussing screening options with your doctor to create a personalized plan based on various risk factors. Here are some questions to help guide your discussion:

1. Family History: Do you have a family history of prostate, ovarian, breast, colon, pancreatic, or other cancers among both male and female relatives? Certain genetic mutations can increase the likelihood of certain cancers. If your family history suggests this, consider discussing screening around age 40.

2. Ethnicity: Are you Black? Black men have a higher risk of developing prostate cancer, often a more aggressive form. Starting the screening discussion around age 40 is recommended for Black men.

3. Age: How old are you? While age alone increases the risk of prostate cancer, without other risk factors, screening discussions typically begin around age 45. As you approach 70 years old, screening recommendations vary. The US Preventive

Services Task Force advises against screening after this age due to the potential risks outweighing the benefits. However, if you're healthy and over 70, it's still worth discussing screening options with your doctor on an individual basis.

Ultimately, the goal of screening is to detect active cancer early for successful treatment, aiming for the longest and healthiest life possible. For low-risk cancers, careful monitoring may be sufficient, with treatment reserved only if necessary.

Diagnosis Test for Prostate Cancer.

Early-stage prostate cancer rarely causes symptoms. As the cancer progresses, you might need to pee more often, or find it harder to completely empty your bladder. It might be painful to pee or to ejaculate, and you might have blood in your semen or pee. You might have pain in your lower back, hip and chest and numbness in your feet and legs. If you have any of these symptoms, it's important to see a healthcare provider right away.

Your provider will start off by asking about your symptoms and your medical history. If they suspect you have cancer, they might do a few different tests, like a prostate exam, to confirm your diagnosis and find out how big and how quickly your cancer is growing (what stage it is). Your provider might also do one or more of these tests:

Diagnostic Procedure

A) Prostate-Specific Antigen (PSA) Test:

What It Measures: PSA is a protein produced by the prostate gland. This test shows if your prostate is making higher-than-normal levels of PSA. Elevated levels may indicate the presence of prostate cancer, but other factors can also influence PSA levels.

How It's Done: A blood sample is taken and analyzed for PSA levels.

Considerations: High PSA levels do not definitively diagnose cancer but may prompt further investigation.

B) Digital Rectal Exam (DRE):

What It Involves: A physical examination where a healthcare provider inserts a gloved, lubricated finger into the rectum to feel the prostate for abnormalities like bumps or hard areas on your prostate gland. They'll do this by inserting a gloved, lubricated finger (digit) into your rectum to reach your prostate.

<u>Purpose</u>: DRE helps assess the size, texture, and presence of lumps or irregularities in the prostate.

<u>Considerations</u>: DRE is often performed in conjunction with the PSA test for a more comprehensive evaluation

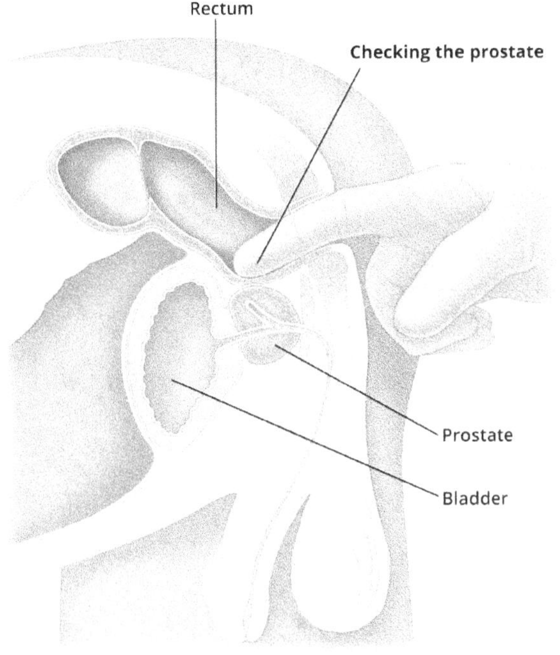

<u>Digital Rectal Exam</u>

<u>C.) Multiparametric Magnetic Resonance Imaging (mpMRI):</u>

<u>What It Involves</u>: Advanced imaging technique using MRI to create detailed images of the prostate.

<u>Purpose</u>: Helps identify suspicious areas that may require further investigation, such as biopsy.

Considerations: mpMRI is increasingly used for targeted biopsies, improving the accuracy of cancer detection.

C) . Genetic Testing:

<u>What It Involves</u>: Analyzing genes associated with an increased risk of prostate cancer, such as BRCA1 and BRCA2.

<u>Purpose</u>: Identifies individuals with a higher genetic predisposition, influencing

screening frequency and potential preventive measures.

Considerations: Genetic testing may be recommended for those with a family history of prostate cancer.

E). Nomograms and Risk Calculators:

What They Are: Tools that estimate an individual's risk of having prostate cancer based on various factors, including age, family history, and PSA levels.

Purpose: Assists in decision-making regarding further diagnostic tests or surveillance.

Considerations: Nomograms provide a personalized risk assessment.

F.) Prostate Biopsy

Your provider will use a needle to take a small amount of tissue from your prostate and send it to the laboratory where a pathologist will look at it under a microscope. A biopsy will tell for sure if you have prostate cancer.

Screening and testing for prostate cancer typically involve a combination of methods aimed at detecting the presence of cancer or assessing the risk of its development.

It's important to note that the decision to undergo screening should be based on informed discussions between individuals and their healthcare providers, taking into account individual risk factors and preferences.

Meet Your Healthcare providers from different specialties, will work closely together to plan your personalized treatment based on your values, priorities, tolerance for side effects and desired quality of life. Your care team could include:

- Urologists.
- Oncologists.
- Radiologists (imaging specialists).
- Pathologists (body tissue specialists).
- Anesthesiologists.
- Social workers.
- Nurse practitioners.
- Physician assistants.

If you are confirmed to have prostate cancer, the health worker will decide what type of treatment (if any) will be the most effective for you. Because prostate cancer grows slowly, you might never need treatment. But if you do, there's good news — most prostate cancers are highly curable. Here are the treatment options your health provider might recommend

1) Watchful Waiting or Active Surveillance

Your doctor may recommend a monitoring approach, either Watchful Waiting or Active Surveillance, to observe your tumor's progression before initiating treatment. Since most prostate cancers progress slowly, some doctors advocate for delaying treatment until the cancer shows signs of growth or causes symptoms. With Watchful Waiting, your doctor will regularly assess your symptoms and overall health. Active Surveillance takes it a step further, incorporating regular tests to closely monitor the cancer's development and adjust treatment plans accordingly."

2) Surgery

Surgery is a viable option if you're in good health and your cancer is localized, meaning it hasn't spread. There are various surgical approaches, including removing just the prostate gland or the gland and surrounding tissue.

Common side effects of surgery include urinary incontinence and erectile dysfunction. However, these issues may resolve on their own, especially bladder control problems. It's essential to discuss the potential risks and benefits with your surgeon beforehand, as they may be able to take steps to preserve the nerves surrounding the prostate and minimize these side effects.

3) Radiation

This treatment uses high-energy beams (similar to X-rays) to kill the cancer. It's often a choice when your cancer is low grade or still only in your prostate. You also might have it after surgery to get rid of any cancer cells left behind. It also helps with cancer that has spread to the bone.

There are two types of radiation therapy: external beam radiation and brachytherapy.

External: A machine outside your body directs rays at the cancer. External beam radiation therapy (EBRT) is the most common type of radiation therapy. EBRT uses CT scans and MRIs to map out the location of the tumor cells and X-rays are targeted to those areas. EBRT treatment is non-invasive and there is no down time or healing time.

Internal (brachytherapy): A doctor does surgery to place small radioactive "seeds" into or near the cancer. Brachytherapy involves placing radiation therapy "seeds" or temporary catheters inside the prostate that emit radiation at a very short distance. It is usually done in one to four treatment sessions depending on the method used.

Sometimes, a mix of both treatments works best.

4) Proton Beam Radiation

This special kind of radiation therapy uses very small particles to attack and kill cancer cells that haven't spread.

5) **Radiopharmaceuticals**

Radiopharmaceuticals, or medicinal radio-compounds, are a group of pharmaceutical drugs containing radioactive isotopes. This form of radiation is used to treat patients diagnosed with castration-resistant metastatic prostate cancer as a method of controlling the disease. The drugs can be taken orally or by injection. In some cases, they may be placed in the prostate itself

6) Hormone Therapy

Prostate cancer cells need male sex hormones, like testosterone, to keep growing. This treatment keeps the cancer cells from getting them. Your doctor might call it androgen deprivation therapy. Some hormone treatments lower the levels of testosterone and other male hormones. Other types block the way those hormones work.

7) Chemotherapy

Drugs that you take by mouth or through an IV travel through your body, attacking and killing cancer cells and shrinking tumors. You might get chemo if the disease has spread outside your prostate and hormone therapy isn't working for you.

8) Immunotherapy

This treatment works with your immune system to fight the disease. It's used to treat advanced prostate cancer

9) Bisphosphonate Therapy

If the disease reaches your bones, these drugs can ease pain and prevent fractures

10) Cryotherapy or Cryosurgery

If you have early prostate cancer, your doctor might choose to kill cancer cells by freezing them. They'll put small needles or probes into your prostate to deliver very cold gasses that destroy the cells.

It's hard to say for sure how well it works. Scientists haven't done much long-term research that focuses on using it to treat prostate cancer. It's usually not the first treatment a doctor recommends

11) **Prostate Cancer Vaccine:**

This personalized treatment harnesses the power of your immune system to target and combat cancer cells. It's most effective when used after hormone therapy has stopped working. While its impact on cancer growth is unclear, research suggests it can help extend the lives of men living with prostate cancer. The vaccine is tailored specifically to each individual, and scientists continue to study its potential in the fight against this disease.

12) High-Intensity Focused Ultrasound

High-intensity focused ultrasound is not a standard in care but is used for patients seeking an option between active surveillance and radical therapy. This device produces sound waves that deliver heat energy to kill cancer cells. It's unclear how well it works, as it hasn't yet been compared with other standard prostate cancer treatments.

CHAPTER 7
Categorizing Prostate Cancer

Categorizing Prostate Cancer: An In-Depth Exploration

Categorizing prostate cancer involves a comprehensive assessment of various factors to determine the extent, aggressiveness, and appropriate management strategies. This extensive exploration delves into the intricate process of categorizing prostate cancer, including staging, grading, and risk stratification. Staging and grading systems offer a comprehensive framework for classifying and understanding prostate cancer. Staging assesses the extent of cancer spread, while grading evaluates the cancer's aggressiveness.

1) TNM Staging System:

Staging assesses the extent of prostate cancer, determining if and how far the cancer has spread beyond the prostate. The TNM system (Tumor, Nodes, Metastasis) is commonly used, providing a standardized framework for categorizing the disease based on tumor size, lymph node involvement, and metastasis

A. **Tumor (T):** Describes the primary tumor's size and extent. Ranges from T1 (confined to the prostate) to T4 (spread to adjacent structures).

B. **Node (N):** Evaluates whether cancer has spread to nearby lymph nodes. N0 indicates no lymph node involvement while N1 suggests regional lymph node metastasis.

C. **Metastasis (M):** Identifies the presence or absence of distant metastases. M0 indicates no distant metastasis, while M1 suggests cancer has spread to distant organs.

2) Grading, Gleason Score and Grouping

The Gleason score is a fundamental component of categorization, assessing the aggressiveness of prostate cancer based on tissue examination. It combines two primary patterns seen in the biopsy specimen, with a higher score indicating a more aggressive tumor.

<u>Grading</u>

Medical pathologists calculate Gleason scores by studying tissue samples under a microscope. If you have prostate cancer, your prostate tissues have cells that are mutating or changing from normal cells to abnormal or cancerous cells.

Early on, cancerous cells can masquerade as healthy cells. Over time, cancerous cells look less like healthy cells. Pathologists grade each tissue sample on a 1 to 5 scale. The lower the grade, the more cancer cells look like normal cells:

- Grade 1: The cancerous cells look a lot like normal cells.
- Grades 2-4: Cancerous cells in the tissue look less like normal cells.
- Grade 5: Cancerous cells look very abnormal.

Each area of prostate cancer may have a different grade, so pathologists pick the two areas that make up most of the cancer. They add the two areas' grades to come up with a Gleason score.

For example, if the largest area with cancer is Grade 3 and the next largest area is

Grade 5, the Gleason score is 8. Any area with a combined Gleason score of 6 or higher is considered cancerous.

Gleason Score

Your Gleason score doesn't rank potential ranges like ranges set for elevated PSA (prostate-specific antigen) tests. Instead, providers break Gleason scores into three categories:

- Gleason 6: The cells look like healthy cells, which is called well differentiated.
- Gleason 7: The cells look somewhat like healthy cells, which is called moderately differentiated.
- Gleason 8, 9 or 10: The cells look very different from healthy cells, which is called poorly differentiated or undifferentiated.

A Gleason score isn't good or bad, per se. Knowing your Gleason score is one way that healthcare providers predict how quickly prostate cancer might grow. Gleason scores range from 6 (low-grade cancer) to 10 (high-grade cancer). Low-grade prostate cancer grows more slowly than high-grade cancer and is less likely to spread (metastasize).

It's important to remember your Gleason score is just one of several pieces of information providers use to plan treatment or set a prognosis. They also consider the results of other tests and more biopsy information. For example, when you had your biopsy, your healthcare provider obtained several samples or cores from your prostate.

They checked how many cores had cancerous cells and whether most of the cells in the cores were cancerous cells. Other factors may include:

- Blood PSA level.
- Digital rectal exam results.
- Imaging test results like ultrasound, magnetic resonance imaging (MRI) or positron emission tomography (PET) scan.
- If there's cancer in both sides of your prostate.
- If prostate cancer spread to other areas of your body.

Gleason scores are a grading system for prostate cancer. Healthcare providers use Gleason score results to set up treatment plans. Gleason scores range from 6 (low-grade cancer) to 10 (high-grade cancer). But numbers don't tell the whole story about your prostate cancer. That story starts with your treatment plan and understanding what to expect from your treatment. Think of your Gleason score and other analysis as the next chapter in your story.

Talk to your healthcare provider any time you have questions about your Gleason score or any other test result. They'll be glad to help you understand what the numbers mean.

Grouping

Grade Group 1-5: Introduced to simplify Gleason Scores into five categories. Grade Group 1 corresponds to Gleason Scores 6 or lower, while Grade Group 5 represents Gleason Scores 9-10.

Gleason scores are a grading system for prostate cancer. Medical pathologists set Gleason scores after studying tissue samples under a microscope. Gleason scores range from 6 (low-grade cancer) to 10 (high-grade cancer). Low grade prostate cancer grows more slowly than high-grade cancer and is less likely to spread (metastasize). **Gleason score** is one of the ways healthcare providers classify prostate cancer as they develop treatment plans or set prognoses (what you can expect after treatment).

Impact on Treatment Decisions:
- Staging and grading inform treatment decisions, helping determine the appropriate interventions based on the cancer's characteristics.
- Treatment may range from active surveillance for low-risk cases to more aggressive approaches for advanced stages.

3) Risk Stratification of Prostate Cancer

Risk stratification is a crucial aspect of managing prostate cancer, guiding clinicians in tailoring treatment strategies based on the likelihood of disease progression and aggressiveness. This comprehensive exploration will delve into the low, intermediate, and high-risk categories, encompassing the parameters used for classification, prognostic factors, and the implications for treatment decisions.

Low, Intermediate, and High Risk Stratification:

Risk stratification categorizes prostate cancer into low, intermediate, and high-risk groups. This assessment considers factors such as PSA levels, Gleason score, and clinical stage. It guides treatment decisions, distinguishing between cases that may benefit from active surveillance, localized interventions, or more aggressive therapies.

High-Risk Prostate Cancer:

a. Clinical Characteristics:

I. High-risk prostate cancer is associated with features indicating a higher likelihood of aggressive behavior.

II. Gleason Score: Often Gleason Score 8 or above, indicating poorly differentiated cancer cells.

III. PSA Level: Elevated PSA levels, frequently exceeding 20 ng/mL.

IV. Clinical Stage: Extensive local involvement or signs of regional lymph node involvement (T3 or T4).

b. Prognostic Implications:

- Unfavorable prognosis with a higher risk of disease progression and metastasis.
- Early and aggressive management is often warranted.

Treatment Considerations:

- Aggressive Treatment: Options may include radical prostatectomy, external beam radiation therapy, and androgen deprivation therapy (ADT).
- Combination Therapies: Some cases may benefit from a multimodal approach, combining surgery, radiation, and systemic therapies.

Intermediate-Risk Prostate Cancer:

a. Clinical Characteristics:

- Intermediate-risk prostate cancer displays features between low and high-risk categories.
- Gleason Score: Often Gleason Score 7, indicating moderately differentiated cancer cells.
- PSA Level: Intermediate PSA levels, typically between 10 and 20 ng/mL.
- Clinical Stage: Extending beyond the prostate capsule but without distant metastasis (T2 or T3).

b. Prognostic Implications:

- Intermediate prognosis with a moderate risk of disease progression.
- Treatment decisions are influenced by factors such as age, overall health, and patient preferences.

c. Treatment Considerations:

- Options include radical prostatectomy, external beam radiation therapy, or brachytherapy.
- Androgen Deprivation Therapy (ADT) may be considered in certain cases.

Low-Risk Prostate Cancer:

a. Clinical Characteristics:

- Low-risk prostate cancer is characterized by features indicating a lower likelihood of aggressive behavior and progression.
- Gleason Score: Typically Gleason Score 6 or below, indicating well-differentiated cancer cells.
- PSA Level: Low PSA levels, often below 10 ng/mL.

☐ Clinical Stage: Limited to the prostate (T1 or T2).

b. Prognostic Implications:

☐ Favorable prognosis with a low risk of disease progression.

☐ Potential for active surveillance as a management strategy, avoiding immediate aggressive treatments.

c. Treatment Considerations:

☐ Active Surveillance: Regular monitoring with PSA tests, digital rectal exams, and periodic biopsies.

☐ Definitive Treatment: If progression is observed during surveillance, interventions such as surgery or radiation therapy may be considered.

risk stratification is integral to the management of prostate cancer, guiding clinicians in selecting appropriate treatments based on the individual characteristics of the disease. The evolving landscape of prostate cancer care, incorporating genomic insights and shared decision-making, underscores the importance of tailoring interventions to optimize outcomes for patients across the spectrum of risk categories.

4) Clinical and Pathological Staging:

Combining clinical and pathological staging provides a comprehensive view. Clinical staging utilizes pre-treatment information, while pathological staging involves post-surgical evaluation. The integration of both aids in refining the categorization and treatment planning.

Clinical Staging:

a. Components:

Prostate-Specific Antigen (PSA) Level: Blood tests measure PSA levels, providing an indication of prostate health.

Digital Rectal Examination (DRE): A physical examination where the healthcare provider assesses the size, shape, and consistency of the prostate through the rectum.

Imaging Studies: Techniques such as transrectal ultrasound, magnetic resonance imaging (MRI), and computed tomography (CT) scans help visualize the prostate and surrounding tissues.

b. TNM System:

- The TNM system classifies tumors based on T (tumor size and extent), N (lymph node involvement), and M (metastasis) categories.

☐ T categories range from T1 (small, confined tumors) to T4 (tumors extending into adjacent structures).

c. Clinical Stage Groups:

☐ Stage I: T1 or T2, low PSA levels, no evidence of spread beyond the prostate.

☐ Stage II: T1 or T2, higher PSA levels, or T3, tumor extends beyond the prostate.

☐ Stage III: T4 or involvement of nearby tissues.

☐ Stage IV: Spread to lymph nodes (N1) or distant metastasis (M1).

d. Limitations:

- Clinical staging may have limitations in accurately assessing the full extent of the disease, particularly regarding lymph node involvement and microscopic spread.

Pathological Staging

a. Components:

- **Gleason Score**: Microscopic examination of prostate tissue assigns a Gleason Score based on the appearance of cancer cells, ranging from 6 (well-differentiated) to 10 (poorly differentiated).

- **Surgical Pathology**: Tissue obtained through biopsy or surgery provides information on the size, location, and characteristics of the tumor.

- **Lymph Node Involvement**: Examining lymph nodes removed during surgery determines if cancer has spread.

b. TNM System: The pathological TNM system refines the clinical staging based on the actual findings from surgery or biopsy. Pathological staging includes additional details on tumor characteristics.

c. Pathological Stage Groups:

Stage I: T1 or T2, Gleason Score 6 or lower, confined to the prostate.

Stage II: T1 or T2, Gleason Score 7, tumor may extend beyond the prostate.

Stage III: T3 or T4, or N1 (lymph node involvement).

Stage IV: M1 (distant metastasis).

d. Prognostic Significance: Pathological staging provides more accurate information for predicting the risk of recurrence and guiding treatment decisions.

<u>Integrating Clinical and Pathological Staging</u>:

a. **Multidisciplinary** **Assessment:** Treatment decisions often involve a multidisciplinary team, considering both clinical and pathological staging. The collaborative approach helps tailor interventions based on the specific characteristics of the disease.

b. Post-Treatment Evaluation: Post-treatment, monitoring PSA levels and potential recurrence is essential to assess treatment efficacy and guide further management.

c. Advances in Imaging: Advanced imaging technologies, such as multiparametric MRI, contribute to improved preoperative staging, aiding in surgical planning.

The combination of clinical and pathological staging provides a comprehensive understanding of prostate cancer, assisting healthcare professionals in determining optimal treatment strategies and offering prognostic insights. Advances in diagnostic tools and collaborative approaches continue to refine the staging process, contributing to more personalized and effective management of individuals with prostate cancer.

5) Localized and Advanced Stages of Prostate Cancer

Prostate cancer classification into localized or advanced stages is pivotal for treatment planning, prognosis, and guiding therapeutic decisions. This extensive exploration will delve into the criteria, diagnostic methods, and implications associated with categorizing prostate cancer into localized and advanced stages.

Localized vs. Advanced Prostate Cancer:

a. Criteria: Prostate cancer is classified into two main categories based on its spread: localized and advanced. Localized prostate cancer is contained within the prostate gland, whereas advanced prostate cancer has spread beyond the prostate to nearby tissues, lymph nodes, or even distant organs, such as bones or other parts of the body."

b. Diagnostic Methods:

PSA Levels: Low to moderately elevated PSA levels may indicate the presence of localized disease.

Gleason Score: Gleason Score 6 or below suggests well-differentiated, less aggressive cancer cells.

Clinical Staging (TNM): T1 or T2 stages, indicating tumors that are still within the prostate.

c. Treatment Options:

Active Surveillance: For low-risk cases, monitoring through regular PSA tests, DRE, and periodic biopsies may be employed.

Definitive Treatments: Options include surgery (radical prostatectomy) and radiation therapy, aiming to eradicate the localized tumor.

d. Prognosis:

- Localized prostate cancer often carries a favorable prognosis, especially when detected early and managed appropriately.

Advanced Prostate Cancer:

a. Criteria: prostate cancer indicates the presence of more aggressive disease with potential spread beyond the prostate.

- May involve invasion into surrounding tissues, lymph node involvement, or distant metastasis.

b. Diagnostic Methods:

PSA Levels: Higher PSA levels, especially in the context of a rising trend, may raise suspicion of advanced disease.

Gleason Score: Scores above 7, indicating more poorly differentiated and aggressive cancer cells.

Clinical Staging (TNM): T3 or T4 stages, lymph node involvement (N1), or distant metastasis (M1).

c. Treatment Options:

Systemic Therapies: Androgen deprivation therapy (ADT) or hormone therapy to suppress testosterone and slow cancer growth.

Chemotherapy: Utilized in certain cases, especially if the cancer has become resistant to hormonal treatments.

Targeted Therapies: Emerging approaches targeting specific pathways involved in cancer progression.

d. Prognosis: Advanced prostate cancer carries a more guarded prognosis due to the potential for metastasis and challenges in complete eradication.

Transition States:

a. Biochemical Recurrence: Some cases may experience a rise in PSA levels after initial treatment, indicating biochemical recurrence. This does not necessarily equate to clinical progression, and decisions about further interventions depend on various factors.

b. Castration-Resistant Prostate Cancer (CRPC): This occurs when prostate cancer progresses despite low testosterone levels achieved through ADT. It also signifies a transition to a more aggressive state, often requiring different treatment modalities.

Challenges and Advances:

a. Imaging Technologies: Advanced imaging, such as multiparametric MRI and positron emission tomography (PET) scans, aids in detecting the extent of disease and guiding treatment decisions.

b. Personalized Approaches: The era of precision medicine involves tailoring treatments based on the molecular characteristics of the cancer, enhancing the ability to address advanced disease.

Therefore, categorizing prostate cancer into localized or advanced stages is pivotal for informing treatment decisions and predicting outcomes. Advances in diagnostic methods and treatment modalities contribute to a more nuanced understanding of the disease, allowing for personalized and effective management strategies tailored to the specific characteristics of each case.

CHAPTER 8
Active Surveillance for Prostate Cancer

Treating prostate cancer is a personalized process, and what works for one man may not work for another. When determining the best course of treatment, your doctor will take several factors into account, including:

- The extent of the cancer (tumor size and spread)
- The cancer's growth rate
- Your age and overall health
- Your individual preferences and values

This tailored approach ensures you receive the most effective and suitable treatment for your unique situation.

Active Surveillance for Prostate Cancer

Active Surveillance (AS) has emerged as a thoughtful and increasingly utilized approach in managing prostate cancer, particularly for cases with low-risk characteristics. This extensive exploration delves into the intricacies of Active Surveillance as a treatment option, covering its principles, patient selection criteria, monitoring protocols, psychological aspects, and the evolving landscape of this conservative management strategy.

Quality of Life Considerations:

Active Surveillance is often associated with a favorable impact on quality of life, as it avoids the potential side effects of immediate treatment. Patients on AS may experience fewer complications related to surgery or radiation, contributing to a better overall quality of life. Active Surveillance prioritizes maintaining the patient's quality of life. By avoiding immediate invasive treatments, individuals on Active Surveillance can maintain normal urinary and sexual function. This approach acknowledges that not all prostate cancers warrant aggressive interventions.

Principles of Active Surveillance:

Active Surveillance is a strategy designed to closely monitor low-risk prostate cancer without immediate intervention. The primary goal is to avoid overtreatment in cases where the cancer is slow-growing and poses a low risk of progression.

Patient Selection Criteria

Candidates for Active Surveillance typically have low-risk prostate cancer, characterized by a Gleason score of 6 or lower, low PSA levels, and limited tumor volume clinical stage T1 or T2 tumors. The decision to pursue AS is individualized, considering the patient's age, overall health, and personal preferences.

Shared Decision-Making: The decision to embark on Active Surveillance is a shared process between the patient and the healthcare team. Detailed discussions about the potential risks and benefits, as well as the psychological impact, help in making informed decisions aligned with the patient's values and preferences.

Patient Adherence and Satisfaction: Patient adherence to Active Surveillance protocols is crucial. Urologists work closely with patients to ensure regular follow-ups and address any concerns. Patient satisfaction with this approach is often high, especially among those who avoid unnecessary side effects associated with more aggressive treatments.

Rationale for Active Surveillance: Active Surveillance is employed for low-risk prostate cancer cases, where the cancer is deemed to be slow-growing and unlikely to cause harm during a patient's natural lifespan. The primary goal is to avoid unnecessary interventions, such as surgery or radiation, that may pose risks of side effects.

Monitoring Protocols: Active Surveillance involves regular monitoring through a combination of PSA tests, digital rectal examinations (DRE), and periodic biopsies. Imaging studies, such as multiparametric MRI, may also be employed to assess any changes in the prostate over time.

Criteria for Transition to Treatment:

Specific triggers may prompt a transition from Active Surveillance to active treatment. These can include changes in PSA velocity, an increase in Gleason score on biopsy, or other indications suggesting a shift from low to higher-risk disease.

Risk Reclassification and Transition to Treatment: If there are indications that the cancer is progressing, such as a rise in

PSA levels or changes in biopsy results, the patient may be reclassified as higher risk. At this point, a transition to more active treatment options, such as surgery or radiation therapy, may be recommended.

Evolving Landscape: Active Surveillance protocols continue to evolve with advancements in imaging and biomarker technologies. Multiparametric MRI is increasingly used to enhance the accuracy of monitoring, providing more detailed insights into the prostate and potentially reducing the need for repeat biopsies.

Advancements in Monitoring Technologies: Ongoing advancements in monitoring technologies, such as improved imaging modalities and biomarker assessments, contribute to refining the Active Surveillance approach. These innovations enhance the precision of risk assessment and further tailor monitoring strategies.

Integration into Multidisciplinary Care: Active Surveillance is an integral part of multidisciplinary prostate cancer care. Collaboration between urologists, oncologists, radiologists, and support staff ensures a holistic approach, considering both the medical and psychosocial aspects of patient care

Psychological Aspects:

Active Surveillance brings unique psychological considerations. Patients may experience anxiety about the uncertainty of cancer progression. Robust support systems, counseling, and clear communication from healthcare professionals play a vital role in addressing these concerns.

Long-Term Outcomes:

Studies evaluating the long-term outcomes of Active Surveillance demonstrate that for appropriately selected patients, the approach is associated with favorable outcomes. Many patients on Active Surveillance may never require definitive treatment, while those who do transition to treatment often do so with curative intent.

Psychosocial Support and Education:

Patients opting for Active Surveillance benefit from comprehensive psychosocial support and education. Urologists and healthcare teams ensure that patients understand the nature of their cancer, the rationale behind Active Surveillance, and the potential risks and benefits. This approach fosters shared decision-making and helps alleviate anxiety.

Facts about active surveillance

Active Surveillance is not a treatment aimed at curing prostate cancer but rather a strategy for monitoring low-risk cases without immediate intervention. The goal of Active Surveillance is to avoid unnecessary treatments, such as surgery or radiation therapy, which can have associated side effects. Instead, it involves regular monitoring through PSA tests, digital rectal exams, and periodic prostate biopsies to track the progression of the disease.

If, during the course of Active Surveillance, there are indications that the cancer is progressing, the healthcare team may reconsider the treatment approach. At that point, a shift to more active treatments, such as surgery or radiation therapy, might be recommended to address the advancing cancer. Active surveillance seeks to balance the potential risks and benefits of treatment, ensuring that patients receive interventions only when necessary.

The decision to transition to a curative treatment depends on the specific characteristics of the cancer, changes in monitoring results, and the collaborative decision-making between the patient and their healthcare team.

The goal of Active Surveillance is to avoid unnecessary treatment in cases where the cancer is low-risk and unlikely to progress significantly. It is not intended as a curative approach but rather a strategy to balance disease control with minimizing treatment-related side effects.

If there is evidence of disease progression or a change in risk factors during Active Surveillance, the healthcare team may consider transitioning to curative treatment options. Common curative treatments for prostate cancer include: Prostatectomy, Radiation Therapy, Cryotherapy, Hormone Therapy, Focal Therapy:

Research and Future Directions:

Ongoing research explores refinements in patient selection, monitoring strategies, and the incorporation of novel biomarkers. The aim is to further optimize Active Surveillance protocols and expand its application to a broader range of patients.

Active Surveillance has emerged as a valuable and patient-centric option for managing low-risk prostate cancer. Balancing the benefits of avoiding immediate treatment-related side effects with the need for vigilant monitoring, Active Surveillance reflects a personalized and evolving approach in the dynamic landscape of prostate cancer care. Continuous research and patient-centered initiatives contribute to the ongoing enhancement of Active Surveillance protocols, shaping the future of prostate cancer management.

Genetic Testing for Prostate Cancer

Groundbreaking research supported by the Prostate Cancer Foundation has revealed that genetic mutations play a role in the development of some prostate cancers. While 5-10% of cases are directly inherited due to specific gene changes passed down from parents to offspring, an additional 10-20% are considered 'familial' - meaning that multiple family members may be affected by cancer, although not necessarily due to specific genetic mutations. These findings have significantly advanced our understanding of prostate cancer's genetic links.

Genes are made of DNA, which is the master "instruction manual" that tells every cell in the body which proteins to make – essentially, the information that each cell needs to do its job. A genetic mutation is a change in part of the normal DNA that makes up a gene. Some mutations are hereditary, meaning that they are passed down from one family member to another. Mutations can also be caused after birth by various lifestyle and environmental factors, such as smoking or the UV rays from the sun.

Genetic mutations can be passed down from father to son, father to daughter, mother to son, or mother to daughter. We now know that some of the same gene mutations that cause prostate cancer can also cause other forms of cancer (such as breast, colon, pancreatic, and others) – and vice versa. Therefore, it can be important to consider genetic testing if you have a history of cancer in your family, even if it's not prostate cancer. This is referred to as genetic testing for an inherited mutation or genetic testing for inherited cancer risk. (You may also hear it called "germline genetic testing.")

The testing itself is a simple saliva or blood test. It is important to consult your doctor and/or a genetic counselor to discuss the risks and benefits of genetic testing. Keep in mind that the testing you can order online is not a substitute for clinical genetic testing through a physician or genetics professional.

All patients with prostate cancer who have certain characteristics are now encouraged to speak to their physician about whether they may need genetic testing for an inherited mutation. These characteristics include: high risk, regional, or metastatic prostate cancer, Ashkenazi Jewish ancestry, family history of cancer risk gene mutations (e.g., BRCA1, BRCA2), or a strong family history of prostate or other cancers.

There is another important reason to ask your doctor about genetic testing. If you have advanced prostate cancer, the results of genetic testing may also help guide your treatment. Medications called PARP inhibitors (olaparib and rucaparib) are FDA-approved for patients with metastatic castration-resistant prostate cancer who also have mutations in certain genes that repair damaged DNA.

Biomarker testing, also known as somatic or tumor testing, is a type of cancer testing that analyzes tumor tissue from biopsy samples or post-prostatectomy specimens. This test examines various cancer characteristics, including gene mutations that may have been inherited or developed during the disease's progression. By identifying these biomarkers, healthcare professionals can gain a deeper understanding of the cancer's behavior and potentially inform treatment decisions.

Someday, genetic testing may be a first step that any doctor takes in diagnosing and treating many different types of disease. As medicine continues to transition towards precision medicine, be prepared to be your own patient advocate: know your family cancer history, and don't be shy about asking your doctor if genetic counseling is right for you.

Genetic testing for inherited cancer risk (sometimes called "germline" genetic testing) can offer powerful insight into your individual risk of developing cancer. Much of the newest research into cancer genetics has focused on identifying inherited changes in genes (mutations) that are associated with development of various types of cancer.

If you have any of the following risk factors, you should discuss them with your doctor and consider genetic testing for inherited cancer risk.

- You are diagnosed with high-risk localized, regional, or metastatic prostate cancer

- A blood relative with a known cancer risk gene mutation, such as a BRCA1/2 mutation or Lynch syndrome

- One relative diagnosed with prostate cancer at age 60 or younger OR with high-risk, regional, or metastatic prostate cancer at any age

- One relative diagnosed with colorectal, endometrial, or breast cancer at age 50 or younger

- One relative diagnosed with male breast cancer, ovarian cancer, pancreas cancer

- Two or more relatives with breast cancer or prostate cancer

- Three or more family members on the same side of the family, with one or more of the following cancers:
    - Endometrial cancer
    - Ovarian cancer
    - Pancreas cancer
    - Colorectal cancer
    - Other cancers, e.g., brain cancer

- Ashkenazi Jewish ancestry

If genetic testing reveals that you or a member of your family have one of these critical mutations, your genetic counselor may suggest "cascade" testing. This is when many members of a family are tested to determine who else may have the mutation. With more information at hand, each member of the family can better understand their particular cancer risk, options for early detection, and how to reduce their risk for various other forms of cancer. The information you learn could save the lives of your brothers and sisters, your parents—and your children

CHAPTER 9

Exploring Prostate Cancer Treatments In Dept

Prostate Cancer shows silent progression from asymptomatic at early Stages to serious complications if the necessary intervention is not administered. Prostate cancer often progresses silently in its early stages, exhibiting minimal to no symptoms. This makes routine screening vital for timely detection. Early detection allows for a broader range of treatment options. When prostate cancer is diagnosed in its early stages, treatment interventions like surgery, radiation therapy, and active surveillance are more viable. These options are often associated with higher success rates and fewer side effects.

Curative Treatments for Prostate Cancer

1. **Prostatectomy (Surgery):** Surgical removal of the prostate gland. The purpose of the procedure is to eliminates the primary tumor and is considered curative if the cancer is confined to the prostate.

2. **Radiation Therapy**: High-energy beams are used to target and kill cancer cells. This radiation Destroys cancer cells and may be employed as external beam radiation or brachytherapy (internal radiation).

3. **Cryotherapy**: Freezing of prostate tissue to destroy cancer cells. Cryotherapy targets and eliminates cancer cells within the prostate.

4. Hormone Therapy: Medications to suppress or block the effects of male hormones. Purpose of hormone therapy is to slow down the growth of prostate cancer cells, often used in combination with other treatments.

5. Focal Therapy: Targeted treatment of specific areas within the prostate. Focal therapy aims to treat localized tumors while preserving healthy prostate tissue.

Each patient's situation is unique, and treatment decisions are tailored to individual circumstances.

Prostatectomy

Prostatectomy is a curative surgical intervention designed to eliminate cancerous tissue within the prostate. The procedure is indicated for localized prostate cancer and may be considered in cases where the cancer is confined to the prostate gland.

Introduction to Prostatectomy:

Prostatectomy is a surgical procedure involving the removal of the prostate gland, commonly employed as a treatment for prostate cancer. This extensive exploration delves into the nuances of prostatectomy, encompassing the different types, surgical techniques, considerations, and postoperative care.

Types of Prostatectomy:

There are several types of prostatectomy, each with its unique approach:

Simple Prostatectomy: Partial removal of the prostate, typically used for benign prostatic hyperplasia (BPH) rather than cancer.

Radical Prostatectomy: Removal of the entire prostate gland, seminal vesicles, and surrounding tissues.

Radical Prostatectomy

During radical prostatectomy, the surgeon removes the entire prostate gland, seminal vesicles, and nearby tissues. Lymph nodes may also be sampled for evaluation. The goal is to achieve complete removal while preserving the surrounding structure

Types of Radical Prostatectomy:
Robotic-Assisted Radical Prostatectomy: Incorporates robotic technology to enhance precision, flexibility, and visualization during the procedure.

Laparoscopic Radical Prostatectomy: Utilizes minimally invasive techniques with smaller incisions and the assistance of a camera for visualization.

Open Radical Prostatectomy: Involves a traditional surgical approach with a single, larger incision.

Indications for Radical Prostatectomy: Radical prostatectomy is typically recommended when prostate cancer is localized and has not metastasized. Factors such as the Gleason score, PSA levels, and clinical stage influence the decision for this surgical intervention.

Preoperative Considerations: Before the surgery, patients undergo a comprehensive evaluation, including imaging studies, blood tests, and discussions about potential risks and benefits. Counseling sessions address expectations, potential side effects, and the impact on urinary continence and sexual function.

Radical Prostatectomy Procedure:

Anesthetic Administration: The patient is placed under general anesthesia.

Incision: Depending on the chosen approach (open, laparoscopic, or robotic-assisted), incisions are made to access the prostate.

Removal of Prostate: The entire prostate gland, along with nearby tissues, is carefully removed. Lymph nodes may also be sampled for evaluation.

Preservation of Nerves: Efforts may be made to preserve nerves responsible for erectile function to minimize the risk of postoperative sexual dysfunction.

Closure: The surgical site is meticulously closed, and drainage tubes may be inserted to manage fluids.

Radical prostatectomy is a significant and effective intervention for localized prostate cancer. Whether performed through an open, laparoscopic, or robotic-assisted approach, the surgery requires careful consideration of individual patient factors. Continuous advancements in surgical technology contribute to optimizing outcomes and preserving the quality of life for individuals undergoing radical prostatectomy.

Simple Prostatectomy:
Simple prostatectomy is a surgical procedure primarily used to treat benign prostatic hyperplasia (BPH), a non-cancerous enlargement of the prostate

gland. Unlike radical prostatectomy, which is employed for prostate cancer, simple prostatectomy involves the removal of only a portion of the prostate gland. This extensive exploration delves into the various aspects of simple prostatectomy, encompassing indications, surgical techniques, considerations, and postoperative care.

Introduction to Simple Prostatectomy: Simple prostatectomy is a surgical intervention designed to alleviate symptoms associated with an enlarged prostate, such as urinary difficulties. It is a common treatment for benign prostatic hyperplasia (BPH), a condition prevalent in aging men.

Indications for Simple Prostatectomy:

Simple prostatectomy is indicated when BPH causes significant urinary obstruction, recurrent urinary tract infections, or fails to respond adequately to conservative treatments. It is not typically employed for prostate cancer.

Preoperative Considerations:

Before the surgery, patients undergo a thorough evaluation, including urodynamic studies, imaging studies, and discussions about potential risks and benefits. Preoperative counseling addresses expectations and potential side effects.

.

Surgical Techniques:

Simple prostatectomy can be performed through different techniques, including:

Robotic-Assisted Simple Prostatectomy:
Incorporates robotic technology for enhanced precision and maneuverability

Laparoscopic Simple Prostatectomy: Utilizes minimally invasive techniques with smaller incisions and a camera for visualization.

Open Simple Prostatectomy: A traditional surgical approach with an incision made in the lower abdomen to access and remove the enlarged part of the prostate.

.

Simple Prostatectomy Procedure:
During the procedure, the surgeon removes the enlarged portion of the prostate, leaving the rest of the gland intact. This allows for relief of urinary obstruction while preserving prostate function.

Advancements in Prostatectomy:

Advances in surgical techniques, including robotic-assisted surgery, have contributed to reduced invasiveness, shorter recovery times, and improved outcomes. Research continues to refine surgical approaches and enhance patient outcomes.

Prostatectomy stands as a cornerstone in the comprehensive treatment of localized prostate cancer. Whether performed through open, laparoscopic, or robotic-assisted techniques, the procedure requires careful consideration of individual patient factors. Advances in surgical technology and postoperative care contribute to optimizing outcomes and preserving the quality of life for individuals undergoing prostatectomy. Continuous research and multidisciplinary collaboration further shape the landscape of prostate cancer treatment, ensuring that prostatectomy remains a vital component in the pursuit of effective, patient-centered care.

Simple prostatectomy is a valuable intervention for managing the symptoms of benign prostatic hyperplasia, providing relief from urinary obstruction. Whether performed through open, laparoscopic, or robotic-assisted techniques, the surgery requires careful consideration of individual patient factors. Continuous advancements in surgical technology contribute to optimizing outcomes and preserving the quality of life for individuals undergoing simple prostatectomy.

HORMONE THERAPY

Hormone Therapy in the Treatment of Prostate Cancer:

Hormone therapy, also known as androgen deprivation therapy (ADT), plays a pivotal role in managing prostate cancer by targeting the male hormones, particularly testosterone, that fuel the growth of prostate cells. This extensive exploration will delve into five key subtopics, providing an in-depth analysis of the mechanisms, indications, types, side effects, and evolving trends in hormone therapy for prostate cancer.

Mechanisms of Hormone Therapy:

Prostate Cancer Cell Suppression:
Deprivation of androgens halts the growth and division of prostate cancer cells.

Mechanisms: Downregulation of androgen receptors, induction of apoptosis, and suppression of cell proliferation.

Clinical Impact: Temporary reduction in tumor size and control of localized disease.

Mechanisms of Hormone Therapy in the Treatment of Prostate Cancer

Hormone therapy, also known as androgen deprivation therapy (ADT), employs various mechanisms to disrupt the growth and proliferation of prostate cancer cells, primarily by targeting the actions of androgens, such as testosterone. This comprehensive examination will delve into two key subtopics, offering an in-depth analysis of both androgen deprivation and the downstream effects on prostate cancer cells.

a. **Androgen Deprivation**: Hormone therapy aims to reduce levels of androgens, primarily testosterone, either by inhibiting production or blocking their effects on prostate cells.

Mechanisms: Orchestrated through surgical castration, medical castration using luteinizing hormone-releasing hormone (LHRH) agonists or antagonists, and anti-androgens.

1. Androgen Deprivation:

a. Inhibition of Testosterone Production: One fundamental approach in hormone therapy involves reducing the production of testosterone, a key androgen that fuels the growth of prostate cancer cells.

Medical Castration: Luteinizing hormone-releasing hormone (LHRH) agonists or antagonists are employed to suppress the production of luteinizing hormone, which in turn leads to decreased testosterone production by the testicles.

Surgical Castration: Orchiectomy, the surgical removal of the testicles, achieves a similar result by eliminating the primary source of testosterone production.

Clinical Impact: Lowering testosterone levels starves prostate cancer cells of the androgen they require for growth, inducing a state of androgen deprivation.

2. Downstream Effects on Prostate Cancer Cells:

a. Inhibition of Androgen Receptor Signaling:

Mechanism: Androgen receptors play a pivotal role in transmitting signals that regulate the growth and survival of prostate cancer cells.

Nuclear Translocation: Upon binding to androgens, the androgen receptor translocates to the nucleus, where it regulates the transcription of genes involved in cell proliferation.

Anti-Androgen Action: By blocking androgen receptor activation, anti-androgens disrupt this signaling pathway, impeding the transcription of genes that support cancer cell survival and proliferation.

Clinical Impact: Suppression of androgen receptor signaling contributes to the inhibition of prostate cancer cell growth and induces apoptotic pathways.

b. Induction of Apoptosis and Cell Cycle Arrest:

Mechanism: Androgen deprivation therapy triggers programmed cell death (apoptosis) and halts the cell cycle, preventing further proliferation of prostate cancer cells.

Caspase Activation: Apoptotic pathways are initiated through the activation of caspases, which orchestrate the systematic dismantling of cancer cells.

Cell Cycle Arrest: Androgen deprivation induces arrest at specific points in the cell cycle, preventing cancer cells from progressing through division.

Clinical Impact: By promoting apoptosis and arresting the cell cycle, hormone therapy contributes to the reduction in tumor size and inhibits the progression of prostate cancer.

b. Blockade of Androgen Receptors:

Mechanism: Anti-androgens act by blocking the binding of androgens, including testosterone and dihydrotestosterone (DHT), to their receptors on prostate cancer cells.

Competitive Binding: Anti-androgens compete with endogenous androgens for binding to androgen receptors, preventing the activation of pathways that drive cancer cell proliferation.

Complementary to Castration: Often used in combination with medical or surgical castration to provide a dual mechanism of androgen deprivation.

Clinical Impact: By obstructing androgen receptor activation, anti-androgens further suppress the signaling cascades that promote prostate cancer growth.

Hormone therapy in the treatment of prostate cancer utilizes a multifaceted approach, targeting androgen production and receptor signaling to disrupt the growth and survival of cancer cells. Understanding the intricacies of these mechanisms is crucial for clinicians and patients, providing insights into the rationale behind hormone therapy and its impact on the management of prostate cancer.

Indications for Hormone Therapy in the Treatment of Prostate Cancer:

Hormone therapy, also known as androgen deprivation therapy (ADT), is a cornerstone in the management of prostate cancer. Understanding the specific indications for initiating hormone therapy is crucial for clinicians in tailoring treatment plans to individual patient needs. This comprehensive examination will delve into three key aspects of the indications for hormone therapy, encompassing its role in locally advanced disease, metastatic prostate cancer, and its utilization in combination with other treatment modalities.

Locally Advanced Prostate Cancer:

Indications: Often used as neoadjuvant or adjuvant therapy in conjunction with radiation or after prostatectomy.

Clinical Impact: Reduces the risk of recurrence and improves overall survival rates.

Hormone therapy is a cornerstone for managing cancers that have extended beyond the prostate capsule.

a. Neoadjuvant Hormone Therapy

Indications: Neoadjuvant hormone therapy is often employed before definitive treatment, such as radical prostatectomy or radiation therapy, in cases where prostate cancer has extended beyond the confines of the prostate.

Goals: Reduction of tumor size and downstaging to facilitate subsequent surgical or radiation interventions.

Clinical Impact: Neoadjuvant hormone therapy aims to enhance the effectiveness of localized treatments and improve the likelihood of achieving complete cancer control.

b. **Adjuvant Hormone Therapy**:

Indications: Adjuvant hormone therapy is utilized after localized treatments like prostatectomy or radiation therapy, particularly in cases with high-risk features.

Clinical Impact: Adjuvant hormone therapy seeks to eradicate residual cancer cells and prevent disease progression after primary interventions.

Goals: Minimization of the risk of cancer recurrence and improvement of overall survival rates.

Metastatic Prostate Cancer:

Hormone therapy is a standard treatment for metastatic prostate cancer.

Indications: Aimed at slowing disease progression and alleviating symptoms associated with advanced stages.

Clinical Impact: Provides palliative relief, extends survival, and enhances quality of life.

b. Salvage Hormone Therapy:

Indications: Salvage hormone therapy is initiated when prostate cancer recurs or progresses despite previous local treatments.

Goals: Delaying disease progression, managing symptoms, and extending survival in the setting of recurrent or persistent metastatic disease.

Clinical Impact: Salvage hormone therapy seeks to control cancer growth and prolong disease stability after initial localized treatments.

a. Initial Treatment for Metastatic Disease:

Indications: Hormone therapy is the primary treatment for metastatic prostate cancer, aiming to control disease progression and alleviate symptoms associated with advanced stages.

Goals: Suppression of androgens to halt cancer cell growth, induce tumor regression, and improve overall survival.

Clinical Impact: Hormone therapy in metastatic disease provides palliative benefits, enhancing quality of life and extending survival.

Combination Therapies:

a. Hormone Therapy with Radiation:

- ☐ **Indications**: Combining hormone therapy with radiation is indicated in cases of locally advanced or high-risk prostate cancer..

- ☐ **Clinical Impact:** The combination approach synergistically targets cancer cells locally, increasing the likelihood of eradicating residual disease.

- ☐ **Goals**: Enhanced local control by sensitizing cancer cells to radiation, reducing the risk of recurrence, and improving overall outcomes

b. Hormone Therapy in Advanced Stages:

Indications: Hormone therapy remains a crucial component in the management of advanced stages, including recurrent or metastatic disease.

Goals: Suppressing androgens to control cancer growth, alleviate symptoms, and extend overall survival.

Clinical Impact: Combining hormone therapy with other modalities, such as chemotherapy or immunotherapy, is explored to optimize treatment outcomes and address the complexities of advanced prostate cancer.

The indications for hormone therapy in prostate cancer are diverse, encompassing neoadjuvant and adjuvant settings for localized disease, primary treatment for metastatic disease, salvage therapy for recurrences, and combinations with other modalities to achieve comprehensive cancer management. Tailoring hormone therapy based on the specific clinical scenario is essential to optimize outcomes and improve the overall care of individuals with prostate cancer.

Types of Hormone Therapy in the Treatment of Prostate Cancer:

Hormone therapy, also known as androgen deprivation therapy (ADT), encompasses various approaches aimed at suppressing the actions of androgens, primarily testosterone, which fuel the growth and proliferation of prostate cancer cells. This extensive exploration will delve into the three main types of hormone therapy used in the treatment of prostate cancer, providing an in-depth analysis of each approach, its mechanisms of action, clinical applications, and potential side efeffects

Three Types of Hormone Therapy includes

c) Anti-Androgens

a.   Luteinizing   Hormone-Releasing Hormone (LHRH) Agonists:

b. LHRH Antagonists:

1. Anti-Androgens:

- **Overview**: Block the binding of androgens to their receptors on prostate cells.

- **Administration**: Administered orally, often used in combination with LHRH agonists or antagonists.

- **Clinical Considerations**: May be prescribed as monotherapy for select cases or as part of combination therapy

a. Mechanism of Action: Anti-androgens function by competitively binding to androgen receptors on prostate cancer cells, thereby blocking the actions of endogenous androgens such as testosterone and dihydrotestosterone (DHT). By inhibiting androgen receptor signaling, anti-androgens disrupt the transcriptional activation of genes involved in cancer cell proliferation and survival.

b. Clinical Applications: Anti-androgens are administered orally in the form of tablets or capsules, offering a convenient route of delivery. They are primarily used in combination with LHRH agonists or antagonists as part of combined androgen blockade (CAB) therapy. Anti-androgens may also be prescribed as monotherapy in select cases, particularly in the setting of biochemical recurrence or localized prostate cancer.

Hormone therapy for prostate cancer encompasses LHRH agonists, LHRH antagonists, and anti-androgens, each offering unique mechanisms of action, clinical applications, and potential side effects. Understanding the nuances of each type of hormone therapy is essential for clinicians in optimizing treatment strategies and mitigating adverse effects while maximizing therapeutic efficacy in the management of prostate cancer.

2) Luteinizing Hormone-Releasing Hormone (LHRH) Agonists:

Overview: Synthetic analogs of LHRH that suppress testosterone production by the testicles.

Administration: Typically administered through injections, either monthly or every three to six months.

Clinical Considerations: Initial testosterone surge before suppression occurs, often mitigated with anti-androgens.

a. Mechanism of Action: LHRH agonists function by initially stimulating the release of luteinizing hormone (LH) from the pituitary gland. Continuous stimulation of

LH receptors leads to downregulation and desensitization of pituitary gonadotropin-releasing hormone (GnRH) receptors, resulting in decreased secretion of LH and follicle-stimulating hormone (FSH). Reduced LH levels subsequently suppress testosterone production by the testes, leading to androgen deprivation and inhibition of prostate cancer cell growth.

b. Clinical Applications: LHRH agonists are administered via subcutaneous or intramuscular injections, typically on a monthly or three to six-monthly basis. They are indicated for both locally advanced and metastatic prostate cancer, serving as the cornerstone of androgen deprivation therapy in these settings. LHRH agonists may be used as monotherapy or in combination with other modalities such as radiation therapy or chemotherapy, depending on the disease stage and patient factors.

3) Luteinizing Hormone-Releasing Hormone (LHRH) Antagonists:

LHRH Antagonists:

- **Overview**: Directly block LHRH receptors, rapidly suppressing testosterone without the initial surge.

- **Administration**: Administered as injections, offering a more immediate reduction in testosterone levels.

- **Clinical Considerations**: Efficacy comparable to agonists but without the initial flare.

a. **Mechanism of Action:** LHRH antagonists directly block the GnRH receptors on the pituitary gland, inhibiting the release of LH and FSH without the initial surge seen with agonists. This rapid suppression of gonadotropin secretion leads to immediate reduction in testosterone levels, achieving androgen deprivation more swiftly than agonists.

b. Clinical Applications: LHRH antagonists are administered via subcutaneous injection, providing a convenient and effective means of achieving rapid androgen deprivation. They are indicated for the treatment of advanced prostate cancer, both in the metastatic and non-metastatic settings. LHRH antagonists may be used as monotherapy or in combination with other treatment modalities, offering an alternative to agonists in certain clinical scenarios.

5. Evolving Trends and Future Directions:

a. Combination Therapies: Investigating the efficacy of combining hormone therapy with other targeted agents.

Trends: Ongoing clinical trials explore the use of hormone therapy alongside immunotherapy, chemotherapy, or novel androgen receptor-targeted agents.

Future Directions: Personalized treatment approaches tailored to individual tumor characteristics.

b. Duration of Hormone Therapy:
Balancing the benefits of prolonged hormone therapy with potential side effects.

Trends: Emerging data guide decisions on the optimal duration, with some cases considering intermittent therapy.

Future Directions: Ongoing research aims to define the ideal duration for different clinical scenarios.

Hormone therapy remains a cornerstone in the multifaceted approach to prostate cancer treatment. Understanding its mechanisms, indications, types, side effects, and the evolving trends in its application provides clinicians and patients with a comprehensive perspective, contributing to informed decision-making and improved outcomes in the management of prostate cancer.

RADIATION THERAPY

Radiation Therapy in the Treatment of Prostate Cancer: Prostate cancer is a prevalent malignancy affecting men worldwide, and radiation therapy stands as a pivotal modality in its comprehensive management. This extensive exploration delves into the multifaceted aspects of radiation therapy, covering its types, treatment planning, side effects, and technological advances.

Types of Radiation Therapy: Three types of radiation therapy in treatment of prostate cancer includes:

- External Beam Radiation,
- Brachytherapy and
- Proton Beam Therapy

External Beam Radiation:
External Beam Radiation in the Treatment of Prostate Cancer: Prostate cancer, a prevalent malignancy affecting men, often necessitates a multidimensional approach for effective management. External Beam Radiation (EBRT) stands out as a

fundamental modality, offering targeted radiation to prostate tumors while sparing surrounding healthy tissues. This approach delivers precisely targeted radiation from outside the body to the prostate. Here, Patients undergo daily sessions over several weeks, ensuring gradual and accurate radiation exposure

The three techniques of external beam radiation includes:

i) Conventional (2D) Radiation Therapy:

ii) Three-Dimensional Conformal Radiation Therapy (3D-CRT):

iii) Intensity-Modulated Radiation Therapy (IMRT):

i) Conventional (2D) Radiation Therapy: Traditional technique utilizing two-dimensional imaging for treatment planning. In this procedure, radiation beams are directed at the prostate from various angles. Using this techniques minimize exposure to healthy tissues.

ii) Three-Dimensional Conformal Radiation Therapy (3D-CRT): Advances from 2D, incorporating 3D imaging to shape radiation beams.

Procedure for 3D-CRT enables precise targeting of the prostate, minimizing irradiation of adjacent structures. **Benefits of 3D-CRT includes**: improved accuracy, reducing side effects compared to conventional techniques.

iii) Intensity-Modulated Radiation Therapy (IMRT):

Employs computer-controlled modulators to vary radiation intensity across multiple beam angles. **This Procedure** Optimized dose distribution, shaping beams to the contours of the prostate. **The Benefits** of this procedure is to enhance precision in delivering higher doses to the tumor while sparing healthy tissues. Generally External Beam Radiation is Effective in treating localized tumors, although potential side effects such as fatigue and urinary changes may arise.

Brachytherapy:

Brachytherapy in the Treatment of Prostate Cancer:

Involves implanting radioactive seeds directly into the prostate tissue.

Seeds emit radiation over time, providing localized treatment with minimal impact on surrounding tissues.

Benefits and Considerations: High dose to the tumor, shorter treatment duration, but potential for urinary and sexual side effects.

A Comprehensive Exploration

Prostate cancer management has evolved, and Brachytherapy, an intricate form of radiation therapy, has emerged as a vital modality in the therapeutic arsenal. This extensive examination delves into the nuanced aspects of Brachytherapy, encompassing its techniques, patient selection, side effects, and the evolving landscape of technological advancements.

1. Techniques of Brachytherapy:

i) Low-Dose Rate (LDR) Brachytherapy:

This Involves the permanent implantation of radioactive seeds directly into the prostate.

Procedure: Seeds emit a continuous, low dose of radiation over an extended period. LDR Provides a localized and sustained dose to the tumor, minimizing impact on surrounding healthy **tissues.**

ii). **High-Dose Rate (HDR) Brachytherapy:** Delivers a high dose of radiation temporarily through catheters inserted into the prostate.

Procedure: Catheters are precisely positioned, and a remote-controlled machine administers the radiation. HDR enables targeted, intensified radiation while minimizing radiation exposure to adjacent structures.

c. **Permanent vs. Temporary Brachytherapy:** LDR Brachytherapy involves permanent seed implantation, while HDR Brachytherapy is temporary.

Procedure: Permanent seeds remain in the prostate, whereas temporary catheters are removed after the treatment session. The choice of either permanent or temporary Brachytherapy depends on patient and tumor characteristics, with both techniques demonstrating efficacy.

2. Patient Selection and Planning:

a. Eligibility Criteria: Suitable for patients with localized prostate cancer, typically with a low or intermediate risk profile.

Selection Factors: Consideration of tumor stage, patient health, and preferences.

Benefits and Considerations: Offers a curative option for eligible patients with favorable risk features.

b. Treatment Planning: Precise planning ensures optimal distribution of radiation to the prostate while sparing nearby structures.

Imaging Techniques: CT and ultrasound assist in visualizing the prostate and guiding seed or catheter placement.

Benefits and Considerations: Tailored plans aim to maximize tumor coverage and minimize radiation to healthy tissues.

c. Combined Modalities: Brachytherapy may be combined with External Beam Radiation for enhanced therapeutic effect.

Procedure: External beam radiation provides supplemental treatment to areas beyond the reach of brachytherapy.

Benefits and Considerations: Comprehensive approach targeting both localized and potentially microscopic disease.

4. Advances in Brachytherapy:

a. **Real-Time Planning and Imaging**: Incorporates real-time planning and imaging during the procedure for enhanced precision. Technological Aspects of Brachytherapy includes advanced imaging modalities that improve seed or catheter placement accuracy.

Clinical Benefits: Improved visualization ensures optimal radiation distribution, reducing the risk of complications.

b. Focal Brachytherapy

Targets specific regions of the prostate, sparing healthy tissue.

Procedure: Involves precise seed placement or catheter positioning based on tumor characteristics.

Benefits and Considerations: Minimizes impact on surrounding structures, potentially reducing side effects.

c. Salvage Brachytherapy:

Utilized in cases of recurrent prostate cancer after initial treatment.

Procedure: Involves implanting additional seeds or delivering a higher dose through catheters.

Benefits and Considerations: Salvage brachytherapy offers a curative option for select patients with recurrent disease.

In conclusion, Brachytherapy serves as a dynamic and effective treatment modality for prostate cancer. The diverse techniques, meticulous patient selection, management of side effects, and ongoing technological advancements collectively contribute to improved outcomes and enhanced quality of life for individuals undergoing brachytherapy for prostate cancer.

c. Proton Beam Therapy:

Utilizes proton beams for precise radiation delivery, minimizing damage to surrounding tissues. It Requires specialized facilities, and the treatment course is similar to external beam radiation.

Benefits and Considerations: Reduced radiation exposure to healthy tissues, though limited availability of proton therapy centers.

Proton Beam Therapy in the Treatment of Prostate Cancer: An In-Depth Analysis

Prostate cancer treatment has witnessed a paradigm shift with the advent of Proton Beam Therapy (PBT), a sophisticated form of radiation therapy. This comprehensive exploration delves into the nuanced aspects of PBT, encompassing its principles, advantages, patient selection, side effects, and the evolving landscape of technological advancements.

1. Principles of Proton Beam Therapy:

a. Particle Physics Basis:

Protons, charged particles, are utilized to deliver precise radiation to cancerous tissues.

Mechanism: Protons deposit their maximum energy at the tumor site, known as the Bragg peak, minimizing damage to surrounding healthy tissues.

Benefits and Considerations: Enhanced precision in targeting tumors, reducing radiation exposure to adjacent organs.

b. Treatment Planning:

Requires meticulous treatment planning to exploit the advantages of proton beams.

Imaging Techniques: CT scans and advanced imaging modalities aid in visualizing the prostate for precise treatment planning.

Benefits and Considerations: Tailored plans aim to maximize tumor coverage while sparing healthy tissues.

Advantages of Proton Beam Therapy:
a. Tissue-Sparing Effect: Protons deposit most of their energy at the tumor site, minimizing damage to healthy tissues.
Clinical Benefits: Reduces the risk of long-term side effects associated with radiation exposure to adjacent structures.
Considerations: Particularly advantageous for tumors located near critical structures.

b. Reduced Radiation to Surrounding Organs:
Proton beams allow for precise control of radiation delivery, sparing nearby organs.
Clinical Benefits: Lower doses to organs such as the bladder and rectum, potentially reducing side effects.

Considerations: May contribute to improved quality of life during and post-treatment.

c. Pediatric Applications:

PBT is particularly beneficial for pediatric patients due to its ability to spare normal tissues.

Clinical Benefits: Reduces the risk of secondary cancers and developmental issues in pediatric populations.

Considerations: Proton therapy is increasingly used in pediatric oncology for various tumor types.

3. Patient Selection and Planning:
a. Eligibility Criteria:

Suitable for a variety of prostate cancer cases, particularly those near critical structures.

Selection Factors: Tumor characteristics, patient health, and preferences are considered.

Benefits and Considerations: Offers a curative option with potential advantages for select patient profiles.

b. Treatment Planning:

Precise planning is crucial to exploit the advantages of proton beams.

Imaging Techniques: CT scans and advanced imaging modalities aid in visualizing the prostate for precise treatment planning.

Benefits and Considerations: Tailored plans aim to maximize tumor coverage while sparing healthy tissues

5. Advances in Proton Beam Therapy:

a. Pencil Beam Scanning: Utilizes narrow proton beams that can be precisely controlled, enhancing treatment precision.

Technological Aspects: Advanced scanning technology allows for detailed modulation of the proton beam.

Clinical Benefits: Improved conformity to tumor shape, reducing exposure to nearby healthy tissues.

b. Integrated Imaging:

Real-time imaging during treatment sessions enhances precision and accuracy.

Technological Aspects: Integration of imaging technologies into treatment machines.

Clinical Benefits: Improved targeting and verification, reducing the risk of errors during treatment.

c. Hypofractionation Protocols:

Investigates the use of fewer treatment sessions with higher doses per session.

Clinical Trials: Ongoing studies explore the efficacy and safety of hypofractionation in prostate cancer.

Considerations: May offer a more convenient treatment schedule for patients.

In conclusion Proton Beam Therapy represents a groundbreaking approach in the management of prostate cancer, capitalizing on its unique physical properties to enhance treatment precision and reduce side effects. The dynamic interplay between particle physics principles, clinical advantages, patient selection criteria, and ongoing technological innovations positions PBT as a forefront modality in the evolving landscape of prostate cancer treatment.

Treatment Planning and Simulation:

a. Imaging and Targeting: Advanced imaging techniques such as MRI and CT aid in precise prostate localization.

Procedure: Simulation sessions determine optimal radiation angles and patient positioning.

Benefits and Considerations: Enhanced targeting reduces damage to adjacent organs, improving treatment accuracy.

b. Dose Calculation and Optimization:

Dosimetrists calculate the radiation dose to ensure maximum tumor exposure.

Procedure: Treatment plans are tailored based on tumor characteristics and proximity to critical structures.

Benefits and Considerations: Optimization aims to maximize cancer cell destruction while minimizing damage to healthy tissue.

c. Treatment Verification:

Daily imaging or monitoring during treatment sessions ensures accurate radiation delivery.

Procedure: Varied verification methods, including image-guided radiation therapy (IGRT) or real-time tracking.

Benefits and Considerations: Reduces the risk of errors, enhancing treatment precision and efficacy.

Treatment Planning and Simulation in Radiation Therapy for Prostate Cancer: An In-Depth Exploration

Effective treatment planning and simulation are critical components of radiation therapy for prostate cancer, ensuring precise delivery of therapeutic doses while minimizing exposure to surrounding healthy tissues. This comprehensive examination delves into the nuanced aspects of treatment planning and simulation, covering techniques, imaging modalities, quality assurance, and the evolving landscape of technological advancements.

Importance of Treatment Planning:

a. Precision in Dose Delivery: Treatment planning aims to maximize radiation to the prostate while sparing nearby critical structures.

Technological Advances: Advanced planning software allows for intricate calculations and optimization.

Benefits and Considerations: Achieving a therapeutic dose to the tumor while minimizing toxicity to adjacent organs.

b. Individualized Patient Plans: Each patient's anatomy and tumor characteristics are unique, requiring personalized treatment plans.

Customization Factors: Consideration of tumor size, location, and proximity to organs at risk.

Benefits and Considerations: Tailored plans optimize treatment outcomes and reduce potential side effects.

Imaging Modalities in Treatment Planning:

a. **Computed Tomography (CT)**: CT scans provide detailed anatomical information for treatment planning.

Procedure: Patients undergo CT simulation in the treatment position to ensure accurate representation.

Benefits and Considerations: Precise visualization aids in delineating the prostate and surrounding structures.

b. Magnetic Resonance Imaging (MRI): MRI complements CT scans, offering superior soft tissue contrast.

Integration in Planning: Fusion of MRI with CT data refines tumor delineation and enhances accuracy.

Benefits and Considerations: Improved visualization of the prostate and nearby organs for more precise planning.

c. Positron Emission Tomography (PET): PET scans may be utilized for functional imaging and to identify areas of increased metabolic activity.

Integration in Planning: Combining PET with CT provides comprehensive information for tumor delineation.

Benefits and Considerations: Helps in identifying areas of potential tumor spread or recurrence.

Simulation Sessions:

a. **Patient Positioning**: Accurate simulation requires patients to be positioned precisely as planned during treatment.

Immobilization Devices: Customized immobilization devices aid in maintaining consistent patient positioning.

Benefits and Considerations: Reproducibility ensures the planned dose is delivered with high precision.

b. **Treatment Fields Definition**: Simulation sessions define the treatment fields, including the angles and depths of radiation beams.

Technological Advances: Three-dimensional planning allows for intricate shaping of treatment fields.

Benefits and Considerations: Ensures optimal coverage of the tumor while minimizing exposure to normal tissues.

Quality Assurance in Treatment Planning:

a. **Plan Verification:** Rigorous checks ensure the accuracy of treatment plans before actual radiation delivery.

Dosimetric Analysis: Verification through dose calculations and measurements using phantoms.

Benefits and Considerations: Prevents errors and guarantees that the planned dose is delivered as intended.

b. **Continuous Adaptation**: Adaptive planning allows for modifications based on changes in tumor size or patient anatomy during treatment.

Imaging During Treatment: Cone-beam CT or other imaging modalities provide real-time data for adaptive planning.

Benefits and Considerations: Maximizes precision and efficacy throughout the course of treatment.

Technological Advances in Treatment Planning:

a. **Intensity-Modulated Radiation Therapy (IMRT)**: IMRT optimizes dose distribution through variable intensity radiation beams.

Technological Aspects: Computer-controlled adjustments during treatment ensure precise dose delivery.

Benefits and Considerations: Enhances conformality to tumor shape, minimizing radiation to healthy tissues.

b. Image-Guided Radiation Therapy (IGRT): IGRT utilizes imaging during treatment sessions to verify and adjust the patient's position.

Technological Advances: Real-time imaging enhances accuracy and allows for immediate adjustments.

Benefits and Considerations: Reduces the risk of errors and improves overall treatment precision.

c. **Proton Beam Therapy Planning**: Treatment planning in proton therapy involves precise calculations to exploit the Bragg peak.

Dosimetric Considerations: Planning aims to maximize proton deposition in the tumor while minimizing exit dose.

Benefits and Considerations: Utilizes proton physics for enhanced precision and reduced toxicity.

Treatment planning and simulation are pivotal in ensuring the success of radiation therapy for prostate cancer. The integration of advanced imaging modalities, rigorous quality assurance measures, and continuous adaptation contribute to the evolving landscape of precision medicine, enhancing treatment outcomes and improving the overall quality of care for individuals undergoing radiation therapy for prostate cancer.

Advances in Radiation Therapy:
a. Image-Guided Radiation Therapy (IGRT): Real-time imaging during treatment sessions for enhanced precision.

Technological Aspects: Integration of imaging technologies into treatment machines.

Clinical Benefits: Improved accuracy in targeting tumors, reducing margins and potential side effects.

b. Intensity-Modulated Radiation Therapy (IMRT):

Variable radiation intensity across multiple beam angles.

Precision Planning: Computer-controlled adjustment of radiation intensity during treatment.

Clinical Benefits: Minimizing radiation exposure to healthy tissues while optimizing tumor dose.

c. Stereotactic Body Radiation Therapy (SBRT):

High doses of radiation delivered in fewer sessions.

Treatment Schedule: Typically completed in 1 to 5 sessions.

Clinical Benefits: Shorter treatment duration with comparable efficacy, especially for localized tumors.

Advances in Radiation Therapy for Prostate Cancer: A Comprehensive Overview

In recent years, significant advancements have transformed the landscape of radiation therapy for prostate cancer, offering enhanced precision, reduced toxicity, and improved treatment outcomes. This extensive exploration delves into the latest innovations and techniques, covering technological advancements, treatment delivery modalities, and evolving paradigms in the management of prostate cancer.

1. Technological Innovations:

a. **Image-Guided Radiation Therapy (IGRT):** Integrates real-time imaging during treatment delivery to ensure accurate tumor targeting.

Advantages: Enhances precision by accounting for daily anatomical variations, reducing margins, and minimizing normal tissue exposure.

Technological Aspects: Cone-beam CT, MRI-guided radiation therapy, and advanced imaging algorithms improve localization and treatment accuracy.

b. **Intensity-Modulated Radiation Therapy (IMRT):** Delivers highly conformal radiation doses by modulating beam intensity across multiple angles.

Advantages: Allows for precise dose sculpting, sparing critical structures while delivering escalated doses to the tumor.

Technological Advances: Volumetric modulated arc therapy (VMAT) and dynamic IMRT techniques further refine dose delivery and treatment efficiency.

c. Stereotactic Body Radiation Therapy (SBRT): Utilizes high-dose radiation delivered in a few fractions to complete treatment within a shorter time frame.

Advantages: Offers comparable oncological outcomes to conventional fractionation with fewer treatment sessions, enhancing patient convenience and resource utilization.

Technological Aspects: Advanced motion management techniques and image guidance ensure accurate delivery despite intrafractional motion.

2. Treatment Delivery Modalities:

a. Proton Beam Therapy (PBT): Utilizes protons' unique physical properties to deliver radiation with superior dose distribution and sparing of healthy tissues.

Advantages: Reduces radiation exposure to surrounding organs, minimizing toxicity and potential late effects.

Technological Advances: Pencil beam scanning and intensity-modulated proton therapy (IMPT) refine dose conformity and enable adaptive planning.

b. Brachytherapy: Involves implanting radioactive sources directly into the prostate gland, delivering high doses of radiation locally.

Advantages: Provides excellent tumor control while minimizing radiation to adjacent tissues, preserving functional outcomes.

Technological Aspects: Real-time planning and image-guided techniques optimize seed or catheter placement, enhancing treatment precision.

3. Evolving Treatment Paradigms:

a.   Hypofractionation: Investigates delivering higher doses per fraction over a shorter treatment course, exploiting prostate cancer's sensitivity to fraction size.

Advantages: Reduces overall treatment time, enhancing patient convenience, and potentially improving tumor control.

Technological Considerations: Advanced planning algorithms ensure safe dose escalation while maintaining normal tissue constraints.

b. Adaptive Radiation Therapy (ART):

Incorporates real-time imaging and plan adaptation to accommodate anatomical changes during the treatment course.

Advantages: Ensures optimal dose coverage despite prostate gland motion or volume changes, reducing the risk of underdosing the tumor or overdosing healthy tissues.

Technological Advances: On-board imaging and automated planning algorithms facilitate seamless plan adaptation throughout treatment.

4. Personalized Approaches:

a. Biomarker-Guided Therapy: Utilizes molecular markers to stratify patients based on their tumor biology and predict treatment response.

Advantages: Enables tailored treatment approaches, optimizing therapy selection, and improving outcomes while minimizing toxicity.

Technological Integration: Next-generation sequencing and multiomic profiling facilitate comprehensive tumor characterization and personalized treatment algorithms.

b. Artificial Intelligence (AI) and Machine Learning: Harnesses AI algorithms to analyze complex clinical data, predict treatment outcomes, and optimize treatment planning.

Advantages: Enhances treatment planning efficiency, automates tasks, and identifies patterns that may guide personalized treatment strategies.

Technological Integration: AI-driven treatment planning systems and predictive models improve treatment decision-making and outcomes.

In conclusion, advances in radiation therapy for prostate cancer have revolutionized treatment approaches, offering unprecedented precision, reduced toxicity, and improved outcomes. The integration of cutting-edge technologies, innovative treatment modalities, and personalized approaches heralds a new era in prostate cancer management, maximizing therapeutic efficacy while enhancing patient experience and quality of life. Continued research and technological innovation will further refine and expand the therapeutic armamentarium, ultimately benefiting patients worldwide.

Radiation therapy plays a crucial role in the multidisciplinary approach to prostate cancer treatment. The diversity of its types, precision in treatment planning, management of side effects, and ongoing technological advancements collectively contribute to improving outcomes and enhancing the quality of life for individuals undergoing radiation therapy for prostate cancer

IMMUNOTHERAPY

Immunotherapy in the Treatment of Prostate Cancer:

Immunotherapy has emerged as a promising frontier in the treatment of prostate cancer, leveraging the body's immune system to recognize and combat cancer cells. This extensive exploration will delve into the mechanisms, current immunotherapeutic approaches, clinical applications, challenges, and future directions in utilizing immunotherapy for prostate cancer.

Mechanisms of Immunotherapy:

a. Immune Checkpoint Inhibition: Immunotherapy often involves targeting immune checkpoints, such as programmed cell death protein 1 (PD-1) and cytotoxic T-lymphocyte-associated protein 4 (CTLA-4). Inhibiting these checkpoints enhances the activation of T cells, promoting an immune response against cancer cells. Checkpoint inhibitors unleash the immune system's potential to recognize and attack prostate cancer cells.

b. Therapeutic Vaccines: Therapeutic vaccines aim to stimulate the immune system to recognize specific antigens on prostate cancer cells. Antigen-presenting cells capture cancer-specific antigens and present them to T cells, triggering an immune response against the tumor. Sipuleucel-T, an FDA-approved therapeutic vaccine, exemplifies this approach in prostate cancer treatment.

Current Immunotherapeutic Approaches:

a. Immune Checkpoint Inhibitors: PD-1/PD-L1 inhibitors (e.g., pembrolizumab, nivolumab) and CTLA-4 inhibitors (e.g., ipilimumab) have been investigated in clinical trials. These agents aim to unleash the immune system by blocking inhibitory signals, promoting T cell activity against prostate cancer cells. Clinical trials explore their effectiveness as monotherapy or in combination with other treatments.

b. Therapeutic Vaccines: Sipuleucel-T, an autologous cellular immunotherapy, involves harvesting a patient's immune cells, exposing them to a prostate cancer antigen, and reinfusing them into the patient. Ongoing research investigates novel vaccine strategies targeting specific prostate cancer antigens to enhance immune responses.

Clinical Applications:

a. Metastatic Castration-Resistant Prostate Cancer (mCRPC): Immunotherapy has shown promise in mCRPC, where conventional treatments may have limited efficacy. Pembrolizumab and nivolumab, PD-1 inhibitors, have been evaluated in clinical trials for their potential in improving outcomes in advanced prostate cancer.

b. Adjuvant and Neoadjuvant Settings: Immunotherapy is explored in combination with standard treatments, such as surgery or radiation, in the adjuvant and neoadjuvant settings. Trials aim to determine the efficacy of boosting the immune response before or after primary interventions.

Challenges in Immunotherapy for Prostate Cancer:

a. Tumor Microenvironment: Prostate cancer often features an immunosuppressive tumor microenvironment, hindering the effectiveness of immunotherapy. Strategies to modify the microenvironment and enhance immune cell infiltration are under investigation.

b. Biomarker Identification:

- Identifying predictive biomarkers for immunotherapy response in prostate cancer remains a challenge.

- Biomarker research focuses on understanding which patients are most likely to benefit from specific immunotherapeutic agents.

Future Directions:

a. Combination Therapies: The future lies in exploring combination therapies, integrating immunotherapy with other modalities like targeted therapies, radiation, or chemotherapy.
Combining different immunotherapeutic approaches may enhance efficacy and broaden the spectrum of responders.

b. Personalized Medicine: Advancements in understanding the unique molecular profiles of prostate cancers may pave the way for personalized immunotherapeutic strategies.
Tailoring treatment based on individual tumor characteristics aims to optimize therapeutic outcomes.

Immunotherapy holds promise in revolutionizing the treatment landscape for prostate cancer. While challenges persist, ongoing research and clinical trials are driving innovation, offering new hope for patients with advanced or aggressive forms of prostate cancer. The dynamic evolution of immunotherapy in prostate cancer underscores the potential for transformative changes in the way we approach and treat this complex disease

Chemotherapy in the Treatment of Prostate Cancer

Chemotherapy, a systemic approach to cancer treatment, plays a distinct role in managing advanced or metastatic prostate cancer. This comprehensive discussion explores the principles, agents, and considerations surrounding chemotherapy for prostate cancer.

Principles of Chemotherapy:

a. Systemic Treatment: Chemotherapy works by targeting rapidly dividing cells throughout the body, aiming to inhibit cancer cell growth.

It differs from localized treatments, such as surgery or radiation, as it addresses cancer cells that may have spread beyond the prostate.

b. Indications: Typically considered in advanced prostate cancer scenarios, especially when the disease is no longer responsive to hormone therapy (castration-resistant prostate cancer, CRPC).

Used to manage symptoms, control disease progression, and potentially extend survival.

Chemotherapeutic Agents:

a. Docetaxel: A taxane chemotherapy drug commonly used in advanced prostate cancer.

 Acts by disrupting microtubule function, inhibiting cell division.

b. Cabazitaxel: Another taxane chemotherapy agent, often considered in cases where docetaxel is no longer effective.

*Provides an alternative mechanism of action.

Combination Therapies:

a. Docetaxel and Hormone Therapy: The combination of docetaxel with hormone therapy has shown improved survival outcomes in certain patient populations.

*Demonstrates the synergy between systemic chemotherapy and androgen deprivation.

b. Sequential Approaches: Some treatment plans involve the sequential use of different chemotherapeutic agents, adapting to the evolving nature of the cancer.

Administration and Monitoring:

a. Intravenous Infusions: Chemotherapy for prostate cancer is typically administered through intravenous infusions. Treatment schedules and dosages are determined based on individual patient factors and response to therapy.

b. Monitoring Response: Regular monitoring, including imaging studies and blood tests, helps assess the response to chemotherapy and adjust treatment plans accordingly.

Advances and Ongoing Research

a. New Agents and Combinations: Ongoing research explores novel chemotherapeutic agents and combination approaches to enhance efficacy and reduce side effects.

b. Precision Medicine: Advances in understanding the molecular landscape of prostate cancer may lead to more targeted and personalized chemotherapy regimens.

In conclusion, chemotherapy represents a valuable tool in the multidisciplinary approach to managing advanced prostate cancer. Its role continues to evolve with ongoing research, emphasizing the importance of individualized treatment plans and a holistic approach to patient care.

CHAPTER 10
SIDE EFFECTS OF PROSTATE CANCER TREATMENTS AND THEIR MANAGEMENT

Prostate cancer treatments can have additional effects on your body beyond just treating the cancer. Potential side effects include:

- Digestive issues
- Decreased libido
- Erectile dysfunction
- Infertility
- Urinary incontinence or frequency

It's essential to consider these side effects when selecting a treatment option. If they become too challenging, you may want to explore alternative approaches. Be sure to discuss your concerns with your doctor, as they can help you anticipate and manage these side effects."

Side Effects of Hormone Therapy:

a. Cardiovascular Risks:

Side Effects: Long-term hormone therapy may increase the risk of cardiovascular issues

Elevated cholesterol levels, increased risk of heart disease, and potential impact on cardiovascular health.

Management: Cardiovascular monitoring, lifestyle modifications, and collaboration with cardiovascular specialists.

b. Bone Health Complications:

Hormone therapy can lead to bone density loss and increase the risk of fractures.

Side Effects: Osteoporosis and fractures, particularly in the hip and spine.

Management: Calcium and vitamin D supplementation, weight-bearing exercises, and bone density monitoring.

Potential Side Effects of Luteinizing Hormone-Releasing Hormone (LHRH)

Common side effects of LHRH agonists include hot flashes, fatigue, decreased libido, erectile dysfunction, and osteoporosis. Initial testosterone surge ("flare reaction") may occur transiently upon initiation of treatment, necessitating concomitant administration of anti-androgens to mitigate symptoms. Long-term use of LHRH agonists may also increase the risk of cardiovascular events and metabolic disturbances.

c. Potential Side Effects: Side effects of LHRH antagonists are similar to those of agonists and include hot flashes, fatigue, sexual dysfunction, and potential bone loss. Compared to agonists, LHRH antagonists may offer a lower risk of testosterone flare, making them preferable in patients with symptomatic or advanced disease.

Potential Side Effects of Anti-androgens
Common side effects of anti-androgens include fatigue, gastrointestinal disturbances, gynecomastia, and sexual dysfunction. Unlike LHRH agonists and antagonists, anti-androgens do not cause testosterone flare, making them suitable for use without concomitant anti-androgen therapy. Long-term use of anti-androgens

may be associated with adverse effects on liver function and potentially cardiovascular health

Side Effects and Management Of Radiation Therapy

Radiation therapy is a cornerstone in the treatment of prostate cancer, effectively targeting cancer cells while aiming to preserve surrounding healthy tissues. However, like any medical intervention, it can induce side effects. This comprehensive examination delves into the nuanced aspects of side effects associated with radiation therapy for prostate cancer, covering short-term and long-term effects, their impact on quality of life, and strategies for effective management.

1. Short-Term Side Effects:

a. Fatigue: Common during and after radiation treatment, impacting energy levels.

Management: Adequate rest, proper nutrition, and moderate exercise can alleviate fatigue.

Impact on Quality of Life: Temporary and often improves post-treatment.

b. Skin Irritation: Localized skin redness or irritation may occur in the treatment area.

Management: Gentle skincare, avoiding harsh products, and following medical advice.

Impact on Quality of Life: Generally temporary and resolves with time.

c. Gastrointestinal Distress: Temporary bowel changes, including diarrhea or urgency.

Management: Dietary modifications, hydration, and medications as prescribed.

Impact on Quality of Life: Often reversible, improving post-treatment.

2. Long-Term Side Effects:

a. Urinary Changes: Irritation or changes in urinary function may persist post-treatment.

Management: Medications, pelvic floor exercises, and lifestyle adjustments.

Impact on Quality of Life: Varied, with some individuals experiencing long-term effects.

b. Sexual Dysfunction: Erectile dysfunction may occur, especially in higher doses or combined therapies.

Management: Medications, counseling, and supportive interventions.

Impact on Quality of Life: Significant and may require ongoing management.

c. Rectal Issues: Long-term rectal irritation or changes in bowel habits.

Management: Dietary adjustments, medications, and ongoing monitoring.

Impact on Quality of Life: Varied, with improvements over time for some individuals.

3. Psychosocial Impact:

a. Anxiety and Depression: A cancer diagnosis and treatment can contribute to emotional distress.

Management: Counseling, support groups, and collaboration with mental health professionals.

Impact on Quality of Life: Recognizing and addressing psychosocial aspects is crucial for overall well-being.

b. Quality of Life Considerations: Cumulative impact of side effects can influence daily life and overall satisfaction.

Management: Comprehensive supportive care, including addressing physical, emotional, and social well-being.

Impact on Quality of Life: Requires a personalized approach, focusing on individual needs and priorities.

4. Late-Onset Side Effects:

a. Radiation Fibrosis: Late tissue scarring in the treated area may occur.

Management: Symptomatic relief, including medications and lifestyle adjustments.

Impact on Quality of Life: Varies, with some individuals experiencing long-term effects.

b. Secondary Cancers: The risk of developing secondary cancers due to radiation exposure.

Management: Ongoing surveillance and early detection strategies.

Impact on Quality of Life: Requires long-term monitoring but can be manageable with timely interventions.

5. Strategies for Effective Management:

a. Multidisciplinary Care: Collaboration between urologists, oncologists, and supportive care teams.

Management: Individualized treatment plans addressing specific side effects and overall well-being.

Impact on Quality of Life: Enhances overall care coordination and patient experience.

b. Supportive Therapies: Integrating complementary therapies, such as physical therapy or acupuncture.

Management: Enhances overall well-being and may alleviate specific side effects.

Impact on Quality of Life: Personalized approaches contribute to a holistic management plan.

c. Survivorship Programs: Long-term care plans addressing post-treatment needs.

Management: Regular follow-up, monitoring, and addressing emerging issues.

Impact on Quality of Life: Empowers survivors with ongoing support and resources.

In conclusion, radiation therapy for prostate cancer is a powerful intervention with potential side effects. Effective management involves a comprehensive, patient-centered approach, addressing short-term and long-term effects through collaboration among healthcare professionals, supportive therapies, and ongoing survivorship programs. Tailoring interventions to individual needs ensures a holistic strategy, promoting the best possible quality of life for individuals undergoing radiation therapy for prostate cancer.

3. Side Effects and Management of Brachytherapy.

a. Short-Term Side Effects: Common effects include temporary urinary changes, mild discomfort, and potential fatigue.

Management: Supportive care measures, including medications to alleviate symptoms.

Impact on Quality of Life: Generally transient, with most side effects resolving post-treatment.

b. Long-Term Side Effects: Potential long-term effects may include urinary changes and, rarely, sexual dysfunction.

Management: Ongoing monitoring and interventions, including medications or lifestyle modifications.

Impact on Quality of Life: Varied, with advancements aiming to minimize long-term effects.

Post-Brachytherapy Imaging: Follow-up imaging, such as MRI or CT scans, assesses treatment response and potential recurrence.

Procedure: Imaging helps evaluate the prostate's condition and identify any areas of concern.

Benefits and Considerations: Monitoring aids in timely interventions if needed and provides reassurance to patients

4. Side Effects and Management:

a. Short-Term Side Effects:

Common effects include temporary fatigue, mild skin irritation, and potential gastrointestinal discomfort.

Management: Supportive care measures, including rest and symptom-specific medications.

Impact on Quality of Life: Generally transient, with most side effects resolving post-treatment.

b. Long-Term Side Effects: Potential long-term effects may include urinary changes and, rarely, sexual dysfunction.

Management: Ongoing monitoring and interventions, including medications or lifestyle modifications.

Impact on Quality of Life: Varied, with advancements aiming to minimize long-term effects.

Side Effects and Management of Radiation therapy

a. Short-Term Side Effects: Common effects include fatigue, skin irritation, and gastrointestinal discomfort.

Management: Supportive care measures, including rest and symptom-specific medications.

Impact on Quality of Life: Generally temporary, with most side effects resolving post-treatment.

b. Long-Term Side Effects:

Potential effects include urinary changes, sexual dysfunction, and the risk of secondary cancers.

Management: Ongoing monitoring and interventions, including medications or lifestyle modifications.

Impact on Quality of Life: Varied, with advancements aiming to minimize long-term effects.

c. Psychosocial Considerations:

Addressing the emotional impact of treatment, including anxiety or depression.

Support Services: Integration of counseling services and support groups.

Impact on Quality of Life: Recognizing and managing psychosocial aspects contributes to overall well-being.

Side Effects and Management of Chemotherapy in Treatments of Prostate Cancer.

a. Hematological Effects: Chemotherapy can impact blood cell production, leading to anemia, neutropenia, or thrombocytopenia. Supportive medications or adjustments in treatment schedules may be employed to manage these effects.

b. Gastrointestinal Issues: Nausea, vomiting, and diarrhea are common side effects. Antiemetic medications and dietary modifications can help alleviate these symptoms.

Patient Considerations:

a. Individualized Decision-Making: The decision to undergo chemotherapy is highly individualized, taking into account factors such as overall health, treatment goals, and patient preferences.

b. Quality of Life: Balancing the potential benefits of chemotherapy with its impact on quality of life is a crucial aspect of treatment discussions.

CHAPTER 11
POST-TREATMENT CARE

Postoperative Care:

After prostatectomy, patients typically stay in the hospital for a brief period. Recovery involves managing pain, monitoring for potential complications, and gradually resuming normal activities. Patients are advised on pelvic floor exercises to support continence and erectile function.

Urinary Continence and Sexual Function: Prostatectomy can impact urinary continence and sexual function. Recovery varies among individuals, and patients are supported through postoperative care, including rehabilitation and discussions about potential interventions for erectile dysfunction.

Follow-Up and Monitoring:

Regular follow-up appointments include PSA tests, digital rectal examinations, and possibly imaging studies to monitor for any signs of recurrence. Ongoing care addresses potential long-term effects and ensures comprehensive postoperative management.

Recovery from Prostate cancer treatment.

Recovery from prostate cancer treatment is a multifaceted journey that varies depending on the individual, the type of treatment received, and other factors such as overall health and lifestyle. While treatment is aimed at eradicating or controlling the cancer, recovery focuses on healing physically, emotionally, and mentally, and returning to a sense of normalcy and well-being.

Physical Recovery:

Physical recovery from prostate cancer treatment can be influenced by the type of treatment undergone. Common treatment options for prostate cancer include surgery, radiation therapy, hormone therapy, chemotherapy, immunotherapy, and active surveillance (watchful waiting). Each of these treatments can have unique physical effects and recovery timelines.

1. Surgery (Prostatectomy):

- Following a prostatectomy, which involves the surgical removal of the prostate gland, recovery typically involves a hospital stay of a few days to a week, depending on the surgical approach (open, laparoscopic, or robotic-assisted).

- Patients may experience pain, discomfort, urinary incontinence, and erectile dysfunction in the immediate postoperative period.
- Recovery involves gradually resuming normal activities, including light exercise and returning to work, under the guidance of healthcare professionals.
- Pelvic floor exercises (Kegel exercises) are often recommended to strengthen the muscles responsible for urinary control.
- Erectile dysfunction may improve over time, but in some cases, it may persist, requiring further treatment such as medication or penile implants.

2. Radiation Therapy:

- Radiation therapy, whether external beam radiation or brachytherapy (internal radiation), can cause side effects such as fatigue, urinary problems, bowel changes, and erectile dysfunction.

- Recovery from radiation therapy involves managing these side effects, which may persist for weeks to months after treatment.

- Patients may benefit from dietary modifications, such as increasing fiber intake to alleviate bowel symptoms, and maintaining hydration to manage urinary symptoms.

- Regular follow-up appointments with healthcare providers are essential to monitor recovery progress and address any lingering side effects.

3. Hormone Therapy:

- Hormone therapy, also known as androgen deprivation therapy (ADT), is often used in combination with other treatments to lower testosterone levels and slow the growth of prostate cancer cells.

- Side effects of hormone therapy may include hot flashes, fatigue, loss of muscle mass, weight gain, and mood changes.

- Recovery from hormone therapy involves managing these side effects through lifestyle modifications, exercise, and supportive care.

- It's important for patients undergoing hormone therapy to maintain regular check-ups with their healthcare team to monitor for potential complications such as osteoporosis or cardiovascular issues.

Emotional and Mental Recovery:

Recovery from prostate cancer treatment also involves addressing the emotional and mental aspects of the journey. A cancer diagnosis and its treatment can evoke a wide range of emotions, including fear, anxiety, sadness, anger, and uncertainty. It's normal for patients to experience these emotions as they navigate the challenges of diagnosis, treatment decision-making, and recovery.

1. Support Groups and Counseling:

- Joining support groups or seeking individual counseling can provide valuable emotional support and coping strategies for patients and their loved ones.
- Talking openly about fears, concerns, and experiences with

others who have gone through similar experiences can help reduce feelings of isolation and provide a sense of belonging and understanding.

☐ Mental health professionals, such as psychologists or social workers, can offer counseling and therapy to help patients cope with emotional challenges and develop healthy coping mechanisms.

2. Lifestyle and Self-Care:

☐ Engaging in self-care activities and maintaining a healthy lifestyle can support emotional well-being and overall recovery.

☐ Regular exercise, such as walking, swimming, or yoga, can help reduce stress, improve mood, and promote physical strength and flexibility.

- ☐ Practicing relaxation techniques, such as deep breathing, meditation, or mindfulness, can help alleviate anxiety and promote a sense of calm and relaxation.

- ☐ Prioritizing sleep and rest is essential for physical and emotional recovery. Establishing a regular sleep schedule and creating a restful sleep environment can improve sleep quality and overall well-being.

3. Open Communication:

- ☐ Open communication with healthcare providers, caregivers, and loved ones is crucial for emotional recovery.

- ☐ Patients should feel comfortable expressing their concerns, asking questions, and seeking support from their healthcare team and loved ones.

- ☐ Loved ones can play a supportive role by listening attentively, offering encouragement and reassurance, and actively participating in the recovery process.

Overall, recovery from prostate cancer treatment is a gradual process that requires patience, perseverance, and a comprehensive approach to physical, emotional, and mental well-being. By taking an active role in their recovery journey and accessing the necessary support and resources, patients can optimize their quality of life and embrace a hopeful future beyond cancer.

CHAPTER 12
Advanced Treatment Options for Prostate Cancer

Advanced treatment options for prostate cancer are constantly evolving, offering patients a range of innovative approaches to effectively manage and combat the disease. These treatments are often tailored to the individual patient's specific diagnosis, stage of cancer, overall health, and treatment goals. The advanced treatments encompass a variety of modalities, including surgery, radiation therapy, hormonal therapy, chemotherapy, immunotherapy, targeted therapy, and emerging techniques such as precision medicine and focal therapy.

Understanding these treatment options is crucial for patients and their healthcare teams to make informed decisions tailored to individual needs and preferences.

1. Targeted Therapy:

Targeted therapy utilizes drugs or other substances to identify and attack specific cancer cells while minimizing damage to healthy cells. These therapies may target proteins, genes, or other molecules that contribute to cancer growth and survival.

Examples of targeted therapies for prostate cancer include:

PARP Inhibitors: These drugs target a specific enzyme involved in repairing damaged DNA, thereby preventing cancer cells from repairing themselves and leading to cell death.

PARP Inhibitors, Poly (ADP-ribose) polymerase (PARP) inhibitors, such as olaparib and rucaparib, target specific genetic mutations in prostate cancer cells, disrupting their ability to repair DNA damage and leading to cell death. These drugs are particularly effective in patients with mutations in the BRCA1, BRCA2, or ATM genes.

Angiogenesis Inhibitors: These drugs block the formation of new blood vessels that supply nutrients to tumors, starving them of essential resources and inhibiting their growth.

2) Immunotherapy:

Immunotherapy works by boosting the body's immune system to recognize and attack cancer cells more effectively. Checkpoint inhibitors, CAR-T cell therapy, and cancer vaccines are among the immunotherapeutic approaches being explored for prostate cancer.

Sipuleucel-T

Sipuleucel-T (Provenge): stimulates the body's immune system to recognize and attack prostate cancer cells. Sipuleucel-T is a personalized immunotherapy that involves harvesting a patient's immune cells, modifying them to target prostate cancer cells, and then infusing them back into the patient to stimulate an immune response.

3. Precision Medicine:

Precision medicine, also known as personalized medicine, involves tailoring treatment strategies based on the unique genetic makeup of each patient's cancer. This approach allows for more targeted and effective therapies, potentially improving treatment outcomes and reducing side effects.

Molecular profiling techniques, such as next-generation sequencing (NGS) and liquid biopsy, are used to analyze tumor DNA and identify specific genetic mutations or alterations that may be targeted with precision therapies.

Precision medicine enables oncologists to select the most appropriate treatment options for individual patients, taking into account factors such as tumor genetics, drug sensitivity, and resistance mechanisms.

Genomic Testing: Genomic testing helps identify specific genetic alterations in a patient's tumor, guiding treatment decisions and personalized therapeutic approaches tailored to the individual's unique cancer profile.

Liquid Biopsies: Liquid biopsies, which analyze circulating tumor cells or cell-free DNA in the blood, provide non-invasive methods for monitoring disease progression, detecting treatment resistance, and guiding targeted therapy selection.

4. Minimally Invasive Surgery:

Minimally invasive surgical techniques, including robotic-assisted laparoscopic surgery, offer patients the benefits of smaller incisions, reduced blood loss, shorter hospital stays, and faster recovery times compared to traditional open surgery.

Robot-assisted radical prostatectomy (RARP) is a commonly performed minimally invasive surgical procedure for the treatment of localized prostate cancer. This approach utilizes robotic technology to enhance surgical precision and dexterity, allowing for more precise tumor removal while preserving surrounding healthy tissue.

Other minimally invasive procedures, such as focal therapy and ablative techniques (e.g Cryotherapy, high-intensity focused ultrasound), target specific areas of the prostate while sparing healthy tissue, minimizing side effects, and preserving quality of life.

Robot-Assisted Radical Prostatectomy (RARP): Robot-assisted surgery, performed using a minimally invasive approach with the assistance of a robotic system, offers several advantages over traditional open surgery, including smaller incisions, reduced blood loss, shorter hospital stays, and faster recovery times.

Nerve-Sparing Techniques: Preservation of the nerves responsible for erectile function during surgery can help minimize the risk of erectile dysfunction following prostatectomy, improving postoperative quality of life for patients.

5. Advanced Radiation Therapy:

Advanced radiation therapy techniques, such as intensity-modulated radiation therapy (IMRT), stereotactic body radiation therapy (SBRT), and proton beam therapy, deliver high doses of radiation precisely to the tumor while minimizing exposure to surrounding healthy tissues.

These techniques allow for more accurate targeting of tumors, improved tumor control rates, and reduced risk of radiation-related side effects.

Image-guided radiation therapy (IGRT) combines real-time imaging with radiation delivery, enabling oncologists to track tumor motion and adjust treatment parameters accordingly, enhancing treatment accuracy and safety.

Stereotactic Body Radiation Therapy (SBRT): SBRT delivers high doses of radiation in fewer sessions than traditional radiation therapy, offering a convenient and effective treatment option for select patients.

Proton Therapy: Proton therapy delivers radiation with pinpoint accuracy, minimizing damage to nearby organs and tissues and reducing the risk of long-term side effects.

6) Hormonal Therapy:

Androgen Deprivation Therapy (ADT): ADT, also known as hormone therapy, suppresses the production of testosterone, a hormone that fuels the growth of prostate cancer cells. It can be used as a standalone treatment or in combination with other therapies to slow disease progression and relieve symptoms.

Second-Line Hormonal Therapies: Novel hormonal therapies, such as enzalutamide and abiraterone, offer additional options for patients with advanced prostate cancer that has become resistant to traditional hormone therapy

:

Docetaxel and Cabazitaxel: Chemotherapy drugs such as docetaxel and cabazitaxel may be used to treat advanced prostate cancer that has spread beyond the prostate and is no longer responsive to hormonal therapy. These drugs work by targeting rapidly dividing cancer cells, slowing tumor growth, and extending survival.

High-Intensity Focused Ultrasound (HIFU) and Cryotherapy: Focal therapy techniques such as HIFU and cryotherapy target and ablate specific areas of the prostate while preserving surrounding healthy tissue, offering a minimally invasive alternative to radical treatments for select patients with localized disease

9). Novel Therapeutic Approaches:

Emerging therapeutic approaches for prostate cancer continue to be investigated in clinical trials, offering promising new treatment options for patients. These include novel drug combinations, gene therapies, RNA-based therapies, and innovative treatment modalities such as nanomedicine and targeted drug delivery systems.

Clinical trials play a critical role in advancing the field of prostate cancer treatment by evaluating the safety and efficacy of these novel therapies and identifying new avenues for improving patient outcomes.

Advancements in prostate cancer treatment are revolutionizing the landscape of care, offering hope for improved outcomes, enhanced quality of life, and prolonged survival for patients. By staying informed about these advanced treatment options and working closely with the healthcare teams, patients can make empowered decisions that align with their individual goals and preferences, ultimately optimizing their journey through prostate cancer treatment and beyond.

CHAPTER 13

CONCLUSION

In closing, "Understanding Prostate Cancer: A Comprehensive Guide to Diagnosis, Treatments, and Recovery" stands as a testament to the empowerment of its readers. Throughout its pages, individuals have been enlightened about the subtle symptoms that may signal prostate cancer's presence, guiding them towards timely diagnosis and intervention.

By delving into the intricacies of diagnosis, the book has armed its audience with the knowledge needed to engage in informed discussions with healthcare professionals, ensuring personalized treatment plans tailored to their unique circumstances.

Furthermore, the book has shed light on the inherent risks and potential side effects associated with various treatment modalities, equipping readers with the tools to navigate these challenges with resilience and grace. Through comprehensive guidance on symptom management and post-treatment care, individuals are empowered to optimize their recovery journey and enhance their overall quality of life.

As readers embark on their respective paths towards healing and renewal, may they carry with them the invaluable insights gleaned from this guide, serving as beacons of hope and empowerment in the face of adversity. With continued advocacy, education, and support, we strive to transform the landscape of prostate cancer care, empowering individuals to live full and vibrant lives beyond their diagnosis.

www.ingramcontent.com/pod-product-compliance
Lightning Source LLC
Chambersburg PA
CBHW051550250726
48653CB00004BA/1076